MANUAL OF GASTROENTEROLOGIC PROCEDURES

Second Edition

Manual of Gastroenterologic Procedures

Second Edition

Editor

Douglas A. Drossman, M.D.
Associate Professor
Division of Digestive Diseases
University of North Carolina School of Medicine
Chapel Hill, North Carolina

Raven Press 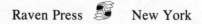 New York

Raven Press, 1185 Avenue of the Americas, New York, New York, 10036

Made in the United States of America

Library of Congress Cataloging-in-Publication Data

Manual of gastroenterologic procedures.

   Includes bibliographies and index.
   1. Gastroenterology—Methodology—Handbooks,
manuals, etc. I. Drossman, Douglas A. [DNLM:
1. Gastroenterology—handbooks. WI 39 M294]
RC802.M35 1987 616.3′3   86-42509
ISBN 0-88167-303-X

9 8 7 6 5 4 3 2 1

This book is dedicated to the memory of Oscar L. Sapp III, M.D., a devoted and respected member of our division for eighteen years. He was an inspiration to those of us fortunate enough to have worked with him.

Preface to the Second Edition

We are pleased to offer a revised procedure manual from our Division of Digestive Diseases at the University of North Carolina School of Medicine. In this edition we continue to present a standardized yet simple approach to learning the indications, contraindications, preparations, techniques, and complications of most all the gastroenterological procedures. As such, it is a resource for physicians, nurses, technicians, and students. The endoscopic chapters provide summary information to supplement some of the more comprehensive manuals recently published. More important, this manual is a unique compendium of all the *nonendoscopic* procedures found within the physician's armamentarium. We know of no other single source that provides "how-to" information for such procedures as nasogastric tube placement; paracentesis; gastric and pancreatic function testing; manometry; small bowel biopsy; liver biopsy; and bougie, wire guide, and balloon dilatation.

We have made several modifications to reflect the rapid changes in gastroenterological practice and technique in the five years since publication of our previous edition. References have been updated and nine new chapters added: the bentiromide test of pancreatic function, balloon (Gruentzig) dilatation of strictures, percutaneous endoscopic gastrostomy (PEG), endoscopic sphincterotomy, coagulation of bleeding gastrointestinal lesions, placement of nasobiliary catheters and endoprostheses, breath H_2 tests, and PH testing for esophageal reflux. The chapter on nasogastric intubation has been expanded to include discussion of the use of small-bore flexible tubes for enteral feeding. The Hollander test (insulin hypoglycemia), having limited diagnostic value and high-risk potential, has been omitted. Finally, a new section addressing the procedural modifications for pediatric patients has been added.

Our publishers tell us that many physicians purchased the previous edition two or three copies at a time. Apparently, they thought the book useful for other members of their staff. We trust that this new edition will continue to serve many purposes for all of us involved in the diagnosis and care of patients with gastroenterological disorders.

Douglas A. Drossman, M.D.

Preface

In recent years, the proliferation of gastroenterologic procedures has broadened the diagnostic and therapeutic options available to the clinician; it has also increased the need for a standardized approach to their selection, technique, and interpretation. Although many textbooks cover the field of gastroenterologic disease, little attention is paid to *how* the morphology and function of the digestive system should be studied. Endoscopy manuals provide extensive detail but do not cover the variety of procedures within the clinician's armamentarium. This volume is the first to present in an organized manner 30 diagnostic and therapeutic procedures frequently used by gastroenterologists, surgeons, and primary care physicians.

The procedural techniques presented and recommendations for use of medication and equipment are those used at the University of North Carolina School of Medicine at Chapel Hill. The reader should consider our suggestions as they pertain to other settings and in the light of the experience of others elsewhere.

Four major areas are discussed: the passage of tubes for measuring intestinal function, endoscopy, diagnosis through the use of percutaneous needle technique, and therapeutic procedures. For quick review, each referenced and illustrated chapter organizes in outline form indications, contraindications, equipment, patient preparation, procedure technique, and interpretation.

The manual cannot teach endoscopy or any other technique that requires supervised training, but it can provide reference criteria for anyone in training. The chapters cover a wide range of procedures—newer, specialized techniques such as rectal manometry and endoscopic sclerosis of esophageal varices, and procedures in common use by primary physicians (nasogastric tube placement, rigid sigmoidoscopy, paracentesis). Also included are some research procedures that might have greater future clinical application (esophageal potential difference measurement, biofeedback for rectal incontinence). Finally, modification of these procedures for use with pediatric patients is included in a separate section.

Douglas A. Drossman, M.D.
1982

Acknowledgments

We would like to thank Peter G. Bedick, Shirley Willard, Sandra Foley Woody, Janet Harris, Gabriel Riggsbee, and Sara Morton for their technical assistance. We would also like to thank Meredith Reinhold and Randy Readling for their assistance in reviewing the manuscript.

Contents

Therapeutic Procedures

Procedures for Pediatric Patients

Contributors

Eugene M. Bozymski, M.D.
Douglas A. Drossman, M.D.
William D. Heizer, M.D.
Ray L. James, Jr., M.D.
Kenneth B. Klein, M.D.
Henry R. Lesesne, M.D.
Sidney L. Levinson, M.D.

C. Thomas Nuzum, M.D.
Roy C. Orlando, M.D.
Don W. Powell, M.D.
Meredith P. Reinhold, R.N.
Robert S. Sandler, M.D.
R. Balfour Sartor, M.D.
Martin H. Ulshen, M.D.

The contributors are members of the Division of Digestive Diseases and Nutrition, School of Medicine, University of North Carolina at Chapel Hill, Chapel Hill, North Carolina. Dr. Ulshen is affiliated with the Department of Pediatrics. All other contributors are affiliated with the Department of Medicine.

The Procedure Unit

Meredith P. Reinhold

Based on our experience at a referral medical center, this chapter offers guidelines for the establishment, organization, and management of a gastrointestinal (GI) procedure unit, many of which can be adapted for use in private practice settings. Its primary focus is creating an environment in which patient needs can be met in a safe, efficient, cost-effective, and concerned manner.

The Procedure Unit

Location and Characteristics

The procedure unit should be located in an area of the hospital readily accessible to both in- and outpatients. The size of the unit and its equipment and furnishings will depend on patient volume and the types of procedures anticipated. Physical separation of the clinical area from the administrative and waiting areas is advisable, and attention should be paid to sound reduction in the clinical areas.

Clinical Area Organization and Equipment (1)

Procedure Rooms

Appropriately furnished procedure rooms should include the following:

1. Contemporary, well-maintained diagnostic and therapeutic instruments with appropriate storage facilities.
2. Movable endoscopy cart.
3. Cleaning facilities, including large sinks, washing, rinsing,

and disinfecting basins, convenient wall suction units, and compressed-air outlet for drying accessories.

4. Wall oxygen, sphygmomanometer.
5. Comfortable, specially designed procedure stretchers with bed-rails and raising, lowering, tilting, and wheel-locking capabilities. If a C-arm fluoroscopy unit will be in use, procedure stretchers should be considered.
6. Intravenous (i.v.) ceiling tracks and hangers.
7. Linen and medication storage areas with locked storage for controlled drugs.
8. Wall-mounted X-ray view boxes.
9. Linen hamper, foot stool, rolling stools, trash receptacle, adequate cabinetry for supplies and accessories, telephone, intercom system, and clock.
10. Provision for patient privacy, adequate ventilation, and lighting with rheostat controls.
11. Allowance for easy transport of stretcher and wheelchair patients.
12. Specimen-handling facilities.
13. Electrocautery equipment.

Accessible Adjuncts to Procedure Rooms

1. Toilet facilities adjoining or adjacent.
2. Clinical sink for disposal of body wastes.
3. Patient dressing area with lockers, toilet, hand-washing sink, linen storage and hamper, sitting bench, call bell, handrails, and wheelchair capacity.
4. Cardiopulmonary resuscitation cart and portable sphygmomanometer.
5. Storage area for traveling endoscopy cart for emergencies.
6. Storage closets for unit supplies and equipment cases.
7. Curtained recovery bed bays or staffed recovery room.
8. Refrigerator for clinical use.
9. Linen supply cart.
10. Patient education room with printed and audiovisual materials and appropriate furnishings.
11. Radiologic facilities within or adjacent to procedure unit.

12. Patient examination room.

Medical Administration Area Organization and Equipment

The allotted space will depend on medical and nursing staffing patterns but should include the following:

1. Medical director's office.
2. Nursing office.
3. Staff physician office space.
4. Staff education room with television monitors and audio equipment, texts, periodicals, and space for unit computer functions.
5. Staff bathroom.
6. Conference and lounge space.
7. Staff refrigerator.
8. X-ray view boxes and film storage units.
9. Dictating and typing equipment.
10. Adequate number of telephone lines, telephones, and an intercom system.

Secretary-Receptionist Area Organization and Equipment

This area should be adjacent to the patient waiting area and readily accessible to the medical staff. Its size depends on the number of personnel, and space must be allotted for the following functions:

1. Patient identification imprinting machine.
2. Computer terminal.
3. Pneumatic tube station.
4. Typewriter.
5. Filing and storage cabinets.
6. Patient record processing.
7. Telephones and intercom controls.
8. Outgoing and incoming mail sorters.
9. Scheduling and patient preparation materials.
10. Storage racks for all pertinent medical forms.

Staff Responsibilities in the Procedure Unit

Medical Staff

1. Provision of consultation services through which the GI procedure unit schedule is generated.
2. Assumption of overall responsibility for medical management and standards of care and for ethical considerations and procedural safety.
3. Maintenance of open lines of communication with nursing and secretarial staff.
4. Teaching designated physicians.
5. Establishment of adequate means of documentation and follow-up.

Nursing Staff

In selecting nursing staff, consideration must be given to the need for administering i.v. medications, to verbal and written communication skills, to the requirement for attention to detail (instrument care), and to coordination skills (instrument handling). Training for work in a GI procedure unit can be accomplished by attending training courses and seminars, supervised on-the-job experience, and familiarization with texts and standardized procedure materials (2). Membership in professional organizations [Society for Gastrointestinal Assistants (SGA) and regional SGA group] is recommended (3).

Patient-Related Responsibilities

The staff's efforts toward patient education, comfort, and emotional support will help ensure a well-accepted and successfully administered procedure. The degree of patient preparation needed will depend on the type of procedure and the needs of the individual patient. All procedures require considerate, individualized attention to the patient by the staff. The following should be accomplished by the nursing staff and/or the physician:

1. Introduce yourself and explain your role in the procedure.
2. After chart review, assess the patient's clinical status, in-

cluding general health and current medications, through questioning and attention to verbal and nonverbal behavior. The patient's ability to understand and communicate and his or her level of apprehension should be noted.

3. Assess the patient's understanding of the procedure.

4. Explain the procedure, keeping in mind your initial assessment of the patient. Patients respond differently in anticipation of unfamiliar, potentially uncomfortable procedures. Some patients benefit from detailed explanations of what to expect, while others do not ask questions and express a desire to "get on with it and get it over with." The latter group may become more agitated if too much effort is made to explain what they would rather not hear (4). In general, a description of the procedure, including sensations likely to be experienced (such as numbness of the throat, a brief needle stick, abdominal cramps), is more valuable than detailed scientific explanations (5,6). The need for the test, alternative therapy, and possible risks and complications should be presented in a straightforward manner. Detailed descriptions of all complications are not necessary (7). It is quite helpful to have available a variety of adjunctive audiovisual materials, including printed patient guides, videotapes, and audio slide equipment, that can be offered to the patient when he or she is confronted with the need for a certain study and again just prior to the actual procedure.

5. Assess the patient's understanding of your explanation and allow sufficient time for questions.

6. Verify written informed consent (8).

7. Ascertain that all the preprocedure requirements have been accomplished by the patient (nothing given by mouth, bowel preparation).

8. Perform the needed preparation [vital signs, draw blood for coagulation studies, subacute bacterial endocarditis (SBE) prophylaxis, start i.v., etc.].

9. During the procedure, monitor the patient's clinical condition (change in vital signs, need for more medication, possible complications), and provide support and reassurance to the patient.

10. At the end of the procedure, reassess the patient's clinical status (e.g., ability to leave the area unattended), and review written postprocedural instructions (possible after-effects and complications, medication schedules, return appointment date) with the patient and family member, if possible. Provide written discharge instructions.
11. Accurately document patient care, responses, and medications on appropriate medical chart forms.
12. Make appropriate patient referrals to Social Work, Home Health, Nutrition Support Team, etc.

Equipment- and Unit-Related Responsibilities

1. Appropriate and meticulous inspection, cleaning, and disinfection of all equipment and accessories immediately after each procedure.
2. Routine maintenance and appropriate storage of all equipment and accessories.
3. Coordination of patient flow and schedule changes with secretary and involved physicians.
4. Provision of written care standards, unit policies, and procedure and job descriptions to ensure continuity and individual and institutional accountability.
5. Maintaining instrument repair records to provide basis for purchase decisions.
6. Adherence to an error-proof system for handling biological specimens.
7. Ordering and distribution of unit supplies, equipment, medications, and linens.
8. Maintaining a procedure complications record as a means of quality assurance (9).
9. Provision of in-service education programs.

Secretarial Staff

As the initial procedure unit contact for patients, and as the persons responsible for schedule organization, the secretary-receptionists play a pivotal role in creating a comforting atmosphere and in fostering the smooth operation of the unit. Their responsibilities include the following:

1. Maintaining the schedule book, which presumes some knowledge of procedure time and room requirements as well as medical-nursing staffing patterns. In a busy referral hospital, this is a singularly complicated assignment.
2. Provision of appropriate medical forms for each case, acquisition and organization of X-ray and laboratory data, and maintenance of patient files and procedure records.
3. Typing and general secretarial duties.
4. Knowledge of medical insurance details.
5. Making appointments and mailing appropriate forms and information.
6. Arranging for patient transportation to and from unit.
7. Being aware of patient needs in waiting area.
8. Labeling and delivery of laboratory specimens.

In conclusion, with the rapid growth of diagnostic and therapeutic procedures in gastroenterology, the goals of safety, efficiency, cost-effectiveness, and considerate patient care can best be met by having adequate staffing and space, open lines of communication, realistic scheduling, and standardized procedural practices where possible.

REFERENCES

1. Standards of Training and Practice Committee, American Society for Gastrointestinal Endoscopy (1980): *Guidelines for the Establishment of a Gastrointestinal Endoscopy Area in Hospitals and Private Offices*. American Society for Gastrointestinal Endoscopy, Boston.
2. Shapiro M, Kuritsky J (1981): *The Gastroenterology Assistant. A Laboratory Manual,* 2nd ed. Valley Presbyterian Hospital, Van Nuys, California.
3. Ravenscroft MM, Swan CHJ (1984): *Gastrointestinal Endoscopy and Related Procedures,* p 1. Williams & Wilkins, Baltimore.
4. Shipley RH, Butt JH, Farbry JE, Horwitz B (1977): Psychological preparation for endoscopy: Physiological and behavioral changes in patients with differing coping styles for stress. *Gastrointest Endosc* 24:9–13.
5. Hartfield MJ, Cason CL (1981): Effective information on emotional responses during the barium enema. *Nurs Res* 30:151–155.
6. Given BA, Simmons SJ (1984): *Gastroenterology in Clinical Nursing,* p 143. CV Mosby Company, St. Louis.

7. Roling GT, Pressgove LW, Keffe EB, Raffin SB (1977): An appraisal of patients' reactions to "informed consent" for peroral endoscopy. *Gastrointest Endosc* 24:69–70.
8. Plumeri DO (1985): Informed consent and the gastrointestinal endoscopist. *Gastrointest Endosc* 31:218–221.
9. Vilardell F (1980): Ethical problems in the management of gastrointestinal patients. *Endoscopy (Suppl)*, 1–12.

1 / Gastrointestinal Intubation

C. Thomas Nuzum and Meredith P. Reinhold

The profusion of pliable, small-bore feeding tubes relegates conventional gastrointestinal tubes to decompression and drainage, gastric lavage, and short-term uses such as diagnostic sampling (1–3). This chapter reviews the characteristics, indications for use, and placement techniques of commonly used tubes.

Indications

In general, the larger caliber polyvinyl tubes are most useful for suction; the thinner silicone and polyurethane tubes are best for long-term infusion. Polyvinyl tubes are also made in small diameter but should be replaced at least weekly because they stiffen with exposure to gastric juice. Use of silicone and polyurethane tubes is relatively free of tissue irritation and pressure necrosis (4). Large-bore orogastric tubes are most effective in removing clots (5).

General Contraindications

1. Nasopharyngeal or upper esophageal obstruction. An alternate entry, such as esophagostomy, gastrostomy, or jejunostomy, may be established.
2. Severe maxillofacial trauma and/or basilar skull fracture.
3. Severe uncontrolled coagulopathy.
4. Varices and severe esophagitis are contraindictions to prolonged use of large-bore polyvinylchloride tubes. Pliability and small diameter reduce trauma and reflux but do not abolish the "wick effect," drawing acid upstream along exterior surface of the tube.

5. Bullous disorders of the esophageal mucosa.

Complications (6–11)

1. Nasal or pharyngeal trauma and hemorrhage.
2. Laryngeal trauma.
3. Laryngotracheal obstruction.
4. Nasotracheal intubation or transbronchial perforation.
5. Pulmonary aspiration.
6. Esophageal and gastric trauma, occasionally leading to hemorrhage or perforation.
7. Intracranial penetration via basilar skull fracture and mediastinal penetration via perforated diverticula are rare mishaps.
8. Chronic irritative complications including rhinitis, pharyngitis, otitis media, esophagitis and gastritis are largely obviated by use of small-bore feeding tubes.

Intubation by Indicated Use

Feeding tubes are discussed here at length. Many of the principles of intubation presented in the first section on feeding tubes apply also to the more familiar tubes described in less detail in the sections on gastric decompression, gastric lavage, and miscellaneous use.

Feeding Tubes
Characteristics (12)

1. 36- to 43-in. long silicone or polyurethane tubes. Transpyloric feedings require 43-in. tubes, which can be utilized for gastric feeding by passing the appropriate length.
2. Intraluminal diameter 5 to 10 French.
3. Distal tip weighted by a tungsten bolus.
4. Placement stylet packaged with tube is also available separately in most cases.
5. Newer products have delivery ports encased in nonperforable material for safer reuse of stylet, if necessary.
6. Radiopaque markings to aid in fluoroscopic placement.
7. Pliability, which increases taping options to the face.

Indications

We assume here a patent gastrointestinal (GI) tract and adequate small bowel absorptive function (13).

1. Inability or unwillingness to ingest sufficient nutrients and/or prescribed medications.
2. Impairment of swallowing or gastric emptying.
3. Need for transition from parenteral to oral alimentation or adjunctive use with limited oral feeding.
4. Need to reduce (but not eliminate) pancreatic or biliary stimulation.

Contraindications (14,15)

1. Complete gastric or intestinal obstruction.
2. Severe gastroesophageal reflux.
3. Ileus.
4. Pancreatic or biliary stimulation undesirable.
5. Patient intolerance to tube.
6. Intractable vomiting.
7. Relative: impaired cough and gag reflexes; mental status changes.

Preparation

1. Read package insert.
2. Give nothing by mouth for several hours if possible because tube passage may provoke vomiting.
3. Explain procedure to patient, including route, purpose, and anticipated duration of intubation.
4. Maintain patient's privacy.

Equipment

1. Appropriate tube and stylet, if necessary.
2. Lubricant, except for tubes with hydromer lubricants.
3. 50-cc Syringe and adapter for irrigating.
4. Semipermeable transparent membrane dressing materials, tincture of benzoin, scissors.
5. 3-cc Syringe for aspiration of gastric contents.

6. Cup of water and straw.
7. Emesis basin and towel.

Procedure

The longer duodenal length tubes can be used for gastric or duodenal placement.

Direct gastric placement

1. Have the patient sit upright, or raise the head of the bed. If this is not possible, a left or right lateral decubitus position has less risk of aspiration than the supine position. Any approach should permit tilting the patient's head forward in the midline.
2. Check for nasal obstruction. Have the patient inhale briskly through each nostril, and use the more patent nostril for intubation.
3. Test the gag reflex. Patients unable to gag are at greater risk of pulmonary aspiration. Local anesthesia is only indicated for the most difficult cases.
4. Estimate length of tube to be inserted. For 90% confidence of placing the tip 1 to 10 cm beyond the cardia in adults, use Hanson's formula (16): (NEX − 50)/2 + 50 cm. Mark the tube 50 cm from its tip. Then, with the patient's head in neutral position, hold the tip of the tube on the patient's nose, and lay the tube along the shortest path from the nose (N) to the earlobe (E) to the xyphoid (X) process. Mark the tube where it reaches the end of the xyphoid. The length of insertion should be halfway between 50 cm and the xyphoid mark. Conventional insertion to the NEX distance placed more than 10 cm of tube in the stomachs of 26% of subjects studied (16). Unless it traverses the pylorus, excess tube in the stomach often loops, pushing the tip into the fundus or cardia.
5. Lubricate tube or activate hydromer lubricant, and examine tube for rough edges or blocked holes. The tube should be emptied of any liquid that might trickle into the trachea. Fix stylet in place if applicable. In more distal placements, removal of the stylet is easier when it has been lubricated.

6. With the patient's neck flexed, gently push the tube through the nares, aiming it back and then down in conformation to the nasopharynx. Pointed too high, the tip will abrade the turbinates. As the tip reaches the posterior pharyngeal wall, have the patient sip water through a straw or initiate dry swallows. This is the most uncomfortable part of the procedure. If resistance is met, retract and try again. Do not force the tube. Endotracheal intubation is usually evinced by the patient's cough and inability to speak, but the smaller tubes do not always elicit these signs. In the unconscious patient, cyanosis may be the first sign of misdirection.
7. Pass tube to predetermined length, checking that it is not coiled in the patient's pharynx and mouth.
8. Confirm passage to stomach by gentle aspiration of gastric contents with a 3-cc syringe and adapter. Verifying tube position by auscultation alone is inadequate. Sounds of air in the bronchial tree have been mistaken for gastric insufflation (7,9,15). Radiologic verification is *mandatory* before feeding is initiated.
9. Tape tube to nose and/or cheek after applying tincture of benzoin. For nose, cut $1\frac{1}{2} \times$ 1-in. piece of nonallergenic tape or semipermeable transparent membrane dressing material. Split one end in half, and place uncut end on patient's nose, wrapping cut ends around tube, being careful to minimize tube contact with nostril.

Placement by gravity into duodenum
1. After gastric placement is verified, place patient on his or her right side for several hours intermittently over the next 24 hr, initially leaving 10 to 20 cm tube slack between tape and nares.
2. Check tube position fluoroscopically. If pyloric passage has not taken place, give Metaclopramide 10 mg i.v. while in fluoroscopy unit. If position is unclear, instill a small amount of dilute contrast material. Irrigate with water after use of contrast material, to avoid clogging.

Endoscopically guided placement into duodenum
Endoscopically guided placement (15) is possible in the presence of esophageal diverticula, strictures, tortuosity, and non-

obstructing lesions. This method also applies to transpyloric placement in the presence of surgical alterations, gastric paresis, and pyloric obstruction.

1. Tie small loop of umbilical tape to distal tip of tube.
2. Pass endoscope into esophagus.
3. Pass lubricated, styleted feeding tube along side of endoscope until loop is visible.
4. Pass grasping forcep through endoscope and grasp loop, guiding feeding tube to appropriate organ.
5. Keep stylet in place until endoscope is removed to prevent friction displacement.
6. Fluoroscopic verification after stylet removal is advised.

Complications

1. Displacement of tube from small bowel to stomach, or from stomach to esophagus, with risk of vomiting and aspiration.
2. Perforation of gut, resulting from misuse or reuse of stylet without fluoroscopy or as a result of overzealous use of a stylet to unclog the tube.
3. Clogging of tube due to inadequate irrigation.
4. Tube rupture as a result of too much irrigation pressure or the use of an irrigation syringe smaller than 50 cc in size (13,15).

Gastric Decompression
Characteristics

1. Length 48 in.; sizes 14, 16, 18 French (also pediatric sizes) polyvinylchloride tubes.
2. Double lumen with radiopaque sentinal line and periodic markings.

Indication

Decompression with gastric atony, ileus, or obstruction.

Procedure

Same as direct placement for feeding tubes, except that no stylet is used. Gastric aspiration is the appropriate placement verification technique.

Gastric Lavage

Characteristics

1. Length, 36 in.; size 34 French, polyvinylchloride or rubber.
2. Large ports.

Indications

1. To empty esophagus or stomach of contents.
2. To irrigate effectively in the presence of bleeding or toxins.

Procedure

1. Explain procedure and place patient in Fowler's or left lateral decubitus position, protected by towels.
2. Pass well-lubricated tube *orally* with neck partially flexed (being cautious to avoid damage to hypopharnyx) and check position before initiating lavage. *Caution:* Release suction and clamp before removing to prevent mucosal trauma and/or aspiration.

Miscellaneous Use

Characteristics

1. Generally 42 to 50 in. in length with a variety of French sizes.
2. Single lumen without radiopaque markings.
3. Least expensive.

Indications

1. Diagnostic sampling (pH, presence of blood).
2. Instillation of medications.
3. Adaptive uses, such as Bernstein and saline load tests.

4. Instillation of balanced electrolyte solutions in whole-gut lavage.

Placement Technique

As in section on gastric decompression.

REFERENCES

1. Cataldo CB, Smith L (1980): *Tube Feedings: Clinical Application.* Ross Laboratories, Columbus, Ohio.
2. Griggs BA, Hoppe MC (1979): Update: Nasogastric tube feeding. *Am J Nurs* 79:481–485.
3. Paine JR (1934): The history of the invention and development of the stomach and duodenal tubes. *Ann Intern Med* 8:752–763.
4. Keoshian LA, Nelson TS (1969): A new design for feeding tube. *Plast Reconstr Surg* 44:508–509.
5. Peterson WL (1983): Gastrointestinal bleeding. In: *Gastrointestinal Disease,* edited by MH Sleisenger, JS Fordtran, p 181. WB Saunders Company Ltd, Philadelphia.
6. Hafner CD, Wylie JS, Brush BE (1961): Complications of nasogastric intubation. *Arch Surg* 83:147–160.
7. Schorlemmer GR, Battaglini JW (1983): An unusual complication of naso-enteral feeding with small diameter feeding tubes. *Ann Surg* 199:104–106.
8. Vaughn ED (1981): Hazards associated with narrow bone nasogastric tube feeding. *Br J Oral Surg* 19:151–154.
9. Hand RW, Kempster M, Levy JH, Rogol PR, Spirn P (1984): Inadvertent transbronchial insertion of narrow-bore feeding tube into the pleural space. *JAMA* 251:239–397.
10. Fremstad J, Martin S (1978): Lethal complication from insertion of nasogastric tube after severe basilar skull fracture. *J Trauma* 18:820–822.
11. Gregory JA, Turner PT, Reynolds AF (1978): Complication of nasogastric intubation: Intracranial penetration. *J Trauma* 18:823–824.
12. Forlaw L, Chernoff R (1984): Enteral delivery systems. In: *Clinical Nutrition, Vol. I,* edited by JL Rombeau and MD Caldwell, pp 228–239. WB Saunders Company Ltd, Philadelphia.
13. Stedman, LW (1984): Nursing aspects of the tube-fed patient. *Nutritional Support Services,* Sept, 36–39.
14. Konstantinides NN, Shronts E (1983): Tube feeding: Managing the basics. *Am J Nurs* 83:1311–1325.

15. Rombeau JL, Jacobs DO (1984): Nasoenteric tube feeding. In: *Clinical Nutrition, Vol I,* edited by JL Rombeau and MD Caldwell, pp 261–274. WB Saunders Company, Ltd, Philadelphia.
16. Hanson RL (1979): Predictive criteria for length of nasogastric tube insertion for tube feeding. *JPEN* 3:160–163.

2 / The Saline Load Test

C. Thomas Nuzum

Gastric emptying is assessed by physical exam (succussion splash), radiography, radioisotope scanning, and intubation studies measuring gastric contents. The saline load test (1) lacks the accuracy, precision, and physiological relevance of infusions employing unabsorbed markers (2) but merits description because of common clinical use.

Indications

1. To test for impaired gastric emptying.
2. To assess healing, efficacy of treatment, and readiness for dietary advancement in patients known to have gastric outlet obstruction and/or disorders of motility.

Contraindications

1. See contraindications to nasogastric intubation (Chapter 1).
2. Small obstructed gastric pouch or voluminous gastroesophageal reflux.
3. Diseases managed by stringent salt and fluid restriction. Water is not substituted for saline because hypotonic duodenal fluid retards gastric emptying (3).

Preparation

1. Nothing by mouth for at least 4 hr.
2. Explain procedure to patient.

Equipment

1. No. 16 French polyvinyl tube with usual accessories for nasogastric intubation (Chapter 1), including "catheter-tipped" 50-cc syringes.
2. Sodium chloride, 750 ml 0.9%, in an open vessel or i.v. infusion set.

Procedure

1. Place the nasogastric tube (Chapter 1).
2. Confirm the tube position radiographically.
3. Aspirate any gastric fluid.
4. Place the patient supine (as originally described) (1) or in left lateral position.
5. Infuse 750 ml saline in less than 5 min from an i.v. set or via syringes.
6. At 30 min, quickly aspirate the gastric contents completely. Obtain as much fluid as possible in the left lateral decubitus, supine, right lateral decubitus, and upright positions. At each position, move the tube in and out over a ±5-cm range.
7. Measure total volume withdrawn in step 6, i.e., the saline residue.

Interpretation

Goldstein and Boyle (1) performed saline load tests in 23 adult men with clinical evidence of gastric retention due to duodenal ulcer (except for two antral cancers) and in 69 control subjects (Table 1). On retesting after 24 hr suction and fluid/

TABLE 1. Original Saline Load Test Results (1)

		Patients (23)	
Control Subjects (69)		Untreated (20)	8–10 hr Nasogastric Suction (3)
Mean residue (ml)	60	640	290
Range (ml)	<200 (63)	370–750	280–295
	205–385 (6)		

electrolyte replacement, 15 of their 23 patients improved, suggesting a reversible component of the obstruction. The authors concluded that "if the initial saline residue is 400 ml or more, it may be said with some confidence that the patient has clinical gastric retention. Values between 300 and 400 ml are suggestive of gastric retention."

The saline load test is not specific for obstruction. Without a marker it fails to distinguish the "retention" of pyloric stenosis from the hypersecretion of Zollinger-Ellison syndrome. Retention occurs in motility disturbances, but because the stomach's emptying rates differ for solid and liquid phases (4,5), a normal liquid residual volume does not rule out disorders like diabetic gastroparesis. The saline load test is of value insofar as it is sensitive to obstruction, simple to perform at the bedside, and cheap. A recent symposium addresses in detail the methodology and interpretation of other gastric-emptying tests (6).

REFERENCES

1. Goldstein H, Boyle JD (1965): The saline load test—a bedside evaluation of gastric retention. *Gastroenterology* 49:375–380.
2. Hunt JN, Knox MT (1968): Regulation of gastric emptying. In: *Handbook of Physiology,* Sect 6, Vol IV, edited by CF Code, pp 1917–1935. American Physiological Society, Washington, DC.
3. Mecroff JC, Go VLW, Philips SF (1975): Control of gastric emptying by osmolality of dudenal contents in man. *Gastroenterology* 68:1144–1151.
4. Pelot D, Dana ER, Berk JE, Dixon G (1972): Comparative assessment of gastric emptying by the "barium-burger" and saline load tests. *Am J Gastroenterol* 58:411–416.
5. Rees WDW, Miller LJ, Malagelada J-R (1980): Dyspepsia, antral motor dysfunction, and gastric stasis of solids. *Gastroenterology* 78:360–365.
6. Dubois A, Castell DO, eds (1984): *Esophageal and Gastric Emptying.* CRC Press, Boca Raton.

3 / Insertion of the Minnesota Tube

Sidney L. Levinson

The Minnesota Four Lumen Esophagogastric Tamponade Tube is used in the treatment of hemorrhage from varices of the esophagus and stomach (1) (Fig. 1). This tube is a new modification of the widely used Sengstaken-Blakemore (SB) tube, incorporating the concept of a separate esophageal suction port (6). Safe use of the SB tube requires ongoing suction of esophageal secretions, and the Minnesota tube contains the port, which in the recent past has had to be applied externally to the SB tube. The new tube has been shown to be better tolerated by patients and easier to use by the staff (1).

The Minnesota tube is used for control of hemorrhage from esophageal varices documented by endoscopy or angiography, which continues despite lavage, correction of blood-clotting abnormalities, and intravenous vasopressin infusion (2–4). The Minnesota tube may be used as an initial measure in patients with life-threatening hemorrhage who have known varices, cirrhosis, or signs of alcoholic liver disease, particularly ascites and jaundice.

Indication

Acute bleeding from esophageal or gastric varices unresponsive to medical therapy.

Contraindications

Absolute

1. Patients in whom variceal bleeding has stopped.
2. Patients with recent surgery involving the esophagogastric junction.

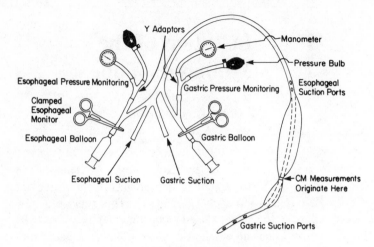

FIG. 1. Minnesota four-lumen tube.

Relative

1. Poorly informed support staff (3).
2. Improper equipment (defective tube, no traction helmet).
3. Congestive heart failure.
4. Respiratory failure.
5. Cardiac arrhythmias.
6. Incomplete lavage.
7. Inability to identify a variceal source of bleeding.
8. Some authors consider a recurrence of bleeding after initial successful tamponade in an operative candidate a relative contraindication (2,4).
9. Esophageal ulceration (secondary to reflux esophagitis or sclerotherapy—in these cases, the gastric balloon may be used but not the esophageal balloon).

Preparation

1. Endoscopy should be performed to confirm the source of bleeding.
2. The staff caring for the patient should have been instructed

in the use of the tube, complications that might arise, and measures for its emergency removal (3).

3. Transfusion with whole blood or blood products should have been instituted.

4. Anesthetize the oropharynx or, if necessary, the nares, with topical agents.

5. With the patient on the left side in semi-Fowler's position, lavage with Adult Gastric Lavage or other large-bore tube using tap water.

6. Test the balloons by insufflating each balloon with air and examining for leaks under water. Connect a mercury manometer to the pressure-monitoring outlet of the gastric balloon. Inflate with increments of 100 cc air and record the corresponding pressure within the gastric balloon.

Equipment

New Minnesota Tube

A commercially available four-lumen tube with aspiration ports in the gastric and esophageal sections, a spherical gastric balloon capable of holding 500 cc air, and a sausage-shaped esophageal balloon with reinforced rubber proximally attached to the gastric balloon. There are ports available for insufflation of the esophageal and gastric balloons and for pressure monitoring of both of these balloons.

Other Equipment

1. Topical anesthesia, such as cetacaine or hurricane spray or diclone gargle, and tongue blades or swabs.

2. Two wall-suction setups with plastic connectors to adapt gastric and esophageal posts to suction tubing.

3. Rubber- or adhesive tape-shod clamps for gastric and esophageal balloon ports.

4. A manometer with pressure bulb attached by connector to one port of the gastric balloon lumen.

5. Water-soluble lubricant.

6. Catheter (60 cc)-tipped syringes.

7. Over-the-bed traction with 1 lb weight is preferred. Helmets or catcher's masks may be used for transportation.

8. Adhesive tape.
9. Scissors, which are to be taped to the head of the bed.

Procedure

1. Suction all air from the balloons and insert plastic plugs.
2. Some authors use intravenous sedation in patients in whom agitation increases the substantial risk of aspiration, and some use atropine to decrease oropharyngeal secretions (4,5). We do not suggest use of sedation or atropine as part of the routine procedure.
3. Clamp rubber-shod clamps on the two pressure-monitoring outlets.
4. Lubricate the tube and pass it through the patient's mouth until the 45-cm mark is located past the dentate ridge. Do not pass the tube through the nares unless orogastric passage is impossible. Since the 45-cm mark is measured from the junction of the esophageal and gastric balloons, patients who are status postgastrectomy may require a different level of placement.
5. Remove the clamps and plastic plugs. Connect the gastric pressure-monitoring outlet to the mercury manometer with a plastic connector. Use the catheter-tip syringe to introduce increments of 100 cc air through the second port, checking manometer readings for correlation with preintubation readings. If the intragastric balloon pressure after intubation is 15 mm Hg greater than that which was produced prior to intubation, then the balloon should be deflated as it is located in the esophagus. The balloon should be deflated immediately if the patient experiences chest pain.
6. When the gastric balloon is inflated with 450 to 500 cc air, clamp the air inlet and pressure-monitoring outlets and pull the tube back gently until resistance is felt against the gastroesophageal junction.
7. Over-the-bed traction set up with 1 lb of weight is recommended. A helmet or mask may be used when the patient is transported.
8. Observe the nature of the drainage from the gastric and

esophageal ports. If bleeding persists from either port, attach the pressure manometer to the esophageal balloon by a Y connector and inflate to a pressure of 25 to 45 mm Hg, using the lowest pressure needed to stop bleeding through both the gastric and esophageal ports. Never inflate the esophageal balloon before the gastric balloon. Double clamp the tube. Periodically check the balloon pressure with the mercury manometer or keep the manometer attached for constant monitoring.

9. Elevate the head of the bed 6 to 10 in. Tape the scissors to the helmet or the head of the bed for quick access in case the balloons need immediate deflation.

Postprocedure

1. Verify the tube position by stat portable X-ray (2,5).
2. Deflate the esophageal balloon for 10 min every 3 hr.
3. Manually check the adequacy of traction at 3-hr intervals. Do not manipulate the tube unnecessarily.
4. Give nothing by mouth. Institute oral hygiene. If necessary, give medicines through the gastric port.
5. Check the gastric and esophageal return regularly and flush both lumens if there is any question of clogging. Barium should never be instilled through the tube, since impaction of balloons could occur, requiring surgical removal of the tube (7).
6. If respiratory distress occurs due to proximal migration of the esophageal balloon with occlusion of the airway, the tube must be removed immediately! *Grasp the tube at the mouth, transect with scissors above the grasping hand but below the entrance of the three channel inlets, and pull out the tube.*
7. If hemostasis persists for 24 hr, deflate the esophageal balloon and release traction. If there is no recurrence of bleeding over the next 6 to 12 hr, deflate the gastric balloon but leave the Minnesota tube in place. If bleeding recurs, the gastric balloon and, if necessary, the esophageal balloon may be reinflated for an additional 24 hr (Fig. 2).
8. Some authors do not suggest a second course of inflation

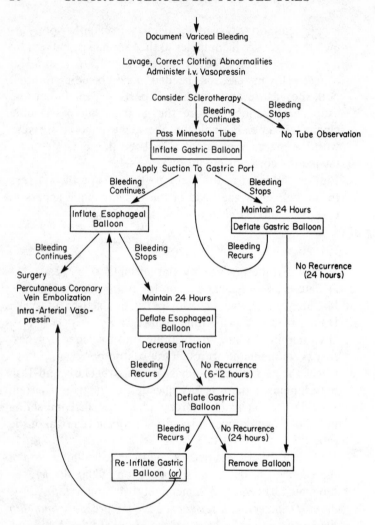

FIG. 2. Therapeutic approach to patient with variceal bleeding.

because of the high mortality rate among patients who rebleed (4). Surgeons should be involved in following the patient.

9. If bleeding does not recur by 24 hr after deflation, remove the Minnesota tube and transect it to ensure that it will not

be reused. This is best done when there is adequate staff available to manage any rebleeding that might occur.

Complications

Major

1. Aspiration. In older series, this was a significant cause of death (2). Aspiration usually occurs during insertion and may occur if the esophageal lumen is obstructed with clots (2,3).
2. Airway occlusion secondary to proximal migration of the tube, which is usually secondary to deflation of the gastric balloon while the esophageal balloon remains inflated (2,3).
3. Pressure effects. Rupture of the esophagus, laceration or ulceration of the stomach, and pressure necrosis of the hypopharynx or alae nasi may occur with prolonged balloon inflation or excessive pressures (2,7). Rupture of the esophagus is a particular risk if sclerotherapy has been performed prior to tube placement.
4. Cardiac arrhythmias.
5. Pulmonary edema.
6. Bronchopneumonia.

Minor

1. Unintentional deflation (3).
2. Inability to deflate because of cementing of the rubber-shod clamps (7).
3. Hiccoughs.
4. Agitation (2,4).

Aspiration, chest pain, and agitation may be decreased if the tube is used without traction.

Efficacy

The Minnesota tube has been shown to be better tolerated than the older SB tubes because of its softer rubber consistency (1). The superior molding of balloons allows for less likelihood of deflation, the ports are better labeled, and aspiration of the esophageal port is easier than the previously modified SB tubes. Although the Minnesota tube can be used safely and may be helpful initially in achieving hemostasis, the final outcome of the patient depends on the level of hepatic function and the development of further episodes of bleeding (4,8).

With proper use of the Minnesota tube, successful tamponade and cessation of bleeding can be achieved in 85% to 92% of patients (1,3,4). In some series, the Minnesota tube is more effective in esophageal variceal bleeding than in gastric variceal bleeding (7). The Minnesota tube is equally effective as i.v. vasopressin in the cessation of esophageal variceal bleeding (9).

The increased usage of esophageal sclerotherapy may alter the use of the Minnesota tube, since sclerotherapy has been shown to be superior to the use of the tube in stopping hemorrhage and in reducing both short- and long-term mortality (10). The use of sclerotherapy carries a 10% complication rate (10). After initial deflation of the Minnesota tube, bleeding may restart in up to 60% of patients (4). In patients who re-bleed when the tube is deflated, the incidence of cessation of bleeding with reinflation falls to 40% to 60% (3,4). In patients with ascites, jaundice, and encephalopathy, the Minnesota tube affords lasting hemostasis in only 25% (4). Without these findings, bleeding does not recur in 92% (4). The overall estimate of achievement of permanent hemostasis is approximately 50% (4,11).

REFERENCES

1. Mitchell K, Silk DB, Williams R (1980): Prospective comparison of two Sengstaken tubes in the management of patients with variceal hemorrhage. *Gut* 21:570–573.
2. Conn HO, Simpson JA (1967): Excessive mortality associated with balloon tamponade of bleeding varices; a critical appraisal. *JAMA* 202:287–291.
3. Pitcher JL Safety and effectiveness of the modified Sengstaken-Blakemore tube: a prospective study. *Gastroenterology* 61:291–298.
4. Novis BH, Duys P, Barbezat GO, et al. (1976): Fiberoptic en-

doscopy and the use of the Sengstaken tube in acute gastrointestinal hemorrhage in patients with portal hypertension and varices. *Gut* 17:258–263.

5. Sengstaken RW, Blakemore AH (1950): Balloon tamponade for the control of hemorrhage from esophageal varices. *Ann Surg* 131:781–789.

6. Boyce HW Jr (1962): Modification of the Sengstaken-Blakemore balloon tube. *N Engl J Med* 267:195–196.

7. Fenig J, Richter RM, Levowitz BS (1976): Gastric ulceration caused by Sengstaken-Blakemore balloon tamponade. *NY State J Med* 76:404–407.

8. Chojkier M, Conn HO (1980): Esophageal tamponade in the treatment of bleeding varices: a decade progress report. *Dig Dis Sci* 25:267.

9. Pinto-Correia J, Martins-Alves M, Alexandrino P, Silveira J (1984): Controlled trial of vasopressin and balloon tamponade in bleeding esophageal varices. *Hepatology* 4:885–888.

10. Paquet KJ, Feussner H (1985): Endoscopic sclerosis and esophageal balloon tamponade in acute hemorrhage from esophagogastric varices: a prospective controlled randomized trial. *Hepatology* 5:580–583.

11. Terblanche J, Yakoob HI, Bornman PC, et al. (1981): Acute bleeding varices: a 5-year prospective evaluation of tamponade and sclerotherapy. *Ann Surg* 195:521.

4 / Esophageal Manometry

Roy C. Orlando

Esophageal manometry is a widely used procedure for the diagnosis and study of esophageal motor disorders (1). The reasons for its popularity are many; among them are the frequency with which patients have symptoms appropriate for study, the ease and safety of performing the test, and the durability and low cost of maintaining the equipment. In recent times, the field of motility has moved from an art to a scientifically based area of investigative work with clinical application (2–4).

Indications

1. To evaluate patients with dysphagia, and/or chest pain for esophageal motor disease.
2. To aid in the diagnosis of progressive systemic sclerosis (scleroderma) or intestinal pseudoobstruction by documenting esophageal motor dysfunction (1).
3. To evaluate the effectiveness of pneumatic dilatation or surgical myotomy in lowering the lower esophageal sphincter pressure (LESP) of patients with achalasia.
4. To evaluate esophageal motility and LESP prior to fundoplication (antireflux surgery) in patients with gastroesophageal reflux and to assess its effectiveness in raising LESP.
5. To localize the lower esophageal sphincter (LES) for positioning of pH probes, perfusion orifices, and biopsy ports.

Contraindications

1. Poor patient cooperation.
2. Patients with cardiac instability or other conditions in which vagal stimulation is poorly tolerated.

Preparation

1. Nothing by mouth for 6 to 8 hr before study.
2. Obtain written consent.

Equipment

1. A triple-lumen polyvinyl catheter assembly (Fig. 1) (internal diameter 1.1 mm) with 1-mm lateral sensing orifices spaced 5 cm apart (Arndorfer Medical Specialties Co., Greendale, Wisconsin). Alternative: Honeywell MP-3 motility probe (Honeywell Biomedical Instrumentation, Denver, Colorado) that contains three miniature pressure transducers.
2. Pneumohydraulic capillary infusion system (Arndorfer Medical Specialties Company, Greendale, Wisconsin)—perfusion rate 0.6 ml/min. Alternative: Harvard pump or

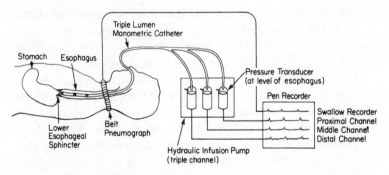

FIG. 1. Performance of esophageal manometry on supine subject using a standard triple-lumen perfused catheter assembly. *Note:* The pressure transducers (more specifically, the diaphragm within the head of the transducer) must be located at the level of the esophagus (midaxillary line) for optimum recording of absolute pressures.

other fluid delivery system with well-greased glass syringes to reduce compliance (2–4).

3. Multichannel recording system (Hewlett Packard Model No. 7758A, Hewlett Packard Company, Palo Alto, California) for use at paper speeds of 1 and 2.5 mm/sec. Alternative: similar equipment available from Beckman Instruments Inc., Schiller Park, Illinois, and Honeywell Biomedical Instrumentation, Denver, Colorado.

4. Pressure transducers for each channel (Model No. 1280-C, Hewlett Packard Company, Palo Alto, California). Alternative: similar equipment available from Beckman Instruments Inc., Schiller Park, Illinois, and Honeywell Biomedical Instrumentation, Denver, Colorado.

5. Swallowing sensor (bellows, sound, or myoelectric type) (Beckman Instruments Inc., Schiller Park, Illinois; Hewlett Packard Co., Palo Alto, California).

6. Catheter-tipped syringe (10–50 cc) for wet swallows.

Procedure[1]

Calibration

1. Calibrate recording system according to manufacturer's directions.

2. Check the accuracy of the fluid-filled pressure transducer and recorder by attaching a sphygmomanometer to each pressure transducer (one at a time or by using an adapter to all three simultaneously) and noting the deflection of the recording needle as the sphygmomanometer is pumped up. *Note.* The needle will respond differently depending on the pressure range selected on the recorder. When testing the system on the 0 to 80 mm Hg scale, pump the sphygmomanometer to approximately 40 mm Hg. The needle should deflect an appropriate number of boxes to reflect this pressure. Repeat this sequence for each pressure range to be used.

3. Following calibration, check the pressure response rate of the system (a measure of its sensitivity to pressure changes

---

[1] For another detailed account see ref. 5 (Chapter 5, pp. 41–51).

within the esophagus) in the following way. Set the recorder on the highest pressure scale and start the fluid delivery pump running at normal speed (0.6 ml/min for Arndorfer pump) with the manometric catheters connected. When water completely fills a catheter and begins to flow from the distal orifice, completely occlude the orifice with your finger. Since the needle deflection produced is a measure of pressure and the paper speed allows a calculation of time, the pressure response rate can be calculated in mm Hg/sec. Response rates ≥150 mm Hg/sec are acceptable for ensuring high-fidelity recordings from the lower and middle third (body) of the esophagus. *Note.* Response rates achievable by perfused catheter systems are inadequate for accurate pressure readings in the upper third (skeletal muscle) of the esophagus, which includes the upper esophageal sphincter. For high-fidelity pressure readings from this area, the Honeywell Model MP-3 motility probe is recommended. The major advantages of perfused catheter systems over the MP-3 motility probe are their flexibility (the number and location of recording orifices can be readily varied—ideal for research) and low replacement costs.

Clinical Study

After calibration, the clinical study is performed by passing the triple-lumen catheter via nose or mouth (nose preferable because of less gagging after passage) into the esophagus (Chapter 1) and advancing it until all channels record gastric pressure. Gastric pressure is indicated by regular low-amplitude waves whose amplitude can be increased by deep inspiration but are unaffected by swallowing (Fig. 2). The absolute gastric pressure usually ranges from 5 to 10 mm Hg when the pressure transducers are correctly located at the level of the esophagus.

Patient Placement

Place the patient in a supine position with arms at sides and attach the swallowing sensor to the neck.

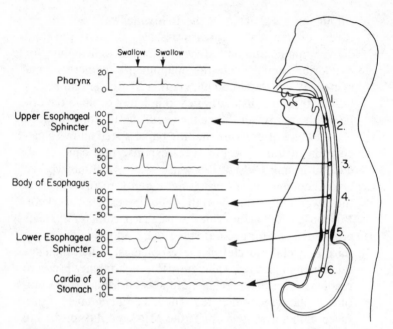

FIG. 2. Schematic representation of the intraluminal pressure events obtained at various points at rest and during swallows in a healthy subject. Pressure scales are in mmHg.

Identify Lower Esophageal Sphincter

With the paper speed set at 1 mm/sec and the recorder on the lowest pressure scale (e.g., 0–80 mm Hg range on Hewlett Packard recorder):

1. Slowly withdraw the catheter assembly until a rise in baseline pressure is noted on the proximal channel. This pressure rise should correspond to the LESP. This is verified by eliciting relaxation with swallows (Fig. 2).
2. Pull-through the LES at ½-cm intervals (station pull-through technique) until all three catheters have traversed it. The LES should appear at each orifice in sequence, approximately 5 cm apart. *Note.* The maximum pressure recorded within the LES may vary considerably for each channel (this reflects differences in spatial orientation of the channels and the asymmetry of the LES muscle). Some

laboratories prefer to use a rapid pull-through technique for obtaining LES pressure (6), though current data do not support this method as being superior to the station pull-through technique. When each channel has passed through the LES, it enters the esophagus.

3. Location of the catheter within the esophagus is indicated by a negative baseline pressure, reflecting intrathoracic pressure, and significant positive pressure waves on swallowing (Fig. 2).

Reposition Catheter Assembly

Reposition the catheter assembly with the distal channel recording from the zone of greatest LES pressure, then fix the assembly in place by taping to the nose. Have the subject swallow two to three times, then adjust the pressure range selector for each channel so that the highest pressures generated remain on scale. Record the proper pressure range for each channel on the manometric paper. Allow 5 min for subjects to adjust to the catheter assembly before formal testing.

Record LES and Esophageal Pressures

Administer a minimum of ten wet swallows (5 cc water given via syringe) at 1- to 2-min intervals. This recording provides information about LES pressure, LES relaxation, peristaltic complexes, and spontaneous contractions in the esophageal body.

After the last wet swallow, remove tape and reposition the catheter assembly with all three channels recording from the esophageal body. This is done by pulling it up 2 to 3 cm above the LES. Retape to the nose.

Perform another 5 to 10 wet swallows in this second position. This recording provides additional information about contractions in the body of the esophagus. In some patients, further sequential withdrawal of the catheter assembly at 1-cm increments, with swallows at each station, can aid in assessing the motor function of the entire esophageal body. This, however, is not generally necessary for diagnosing a motor disorder in most patients.

Upper Esophageal Sphincter

1. Remove tape and slowly withdraw the catheter assembly until the proximal channel encounters another high pressure zone; this is the upper esophageal sphincter (UES). The UES can be verified by eliciting relaxation with swallows, similar to that seen with the LES.
2. Stop perfusion of the proximal channel. This helps to avoid minor aspiration and coughing. Continue the station pull-through until the middle channel records the UES. The proximal channel is now recording pharyngeal contractions and the distal channel is recording from the upper portion of the esophagus.
3. Switch the paper speed to 2.5 mm/sec. (This spreads the complexes, allowing coordination between UES relaxation and pharyngeal contraction to be more easily determined.)
4. With the catheter assembly fixed in this third position, perform 5 to 10 "dry" swallows.

Provocative Testing

For selected patients with unexplained chest pain and/or dysphagia, provocative testing may aid in the diagnosis of symptomatic esophageal motor disease. Such testing is appropriate (a) when routine esophageal manometric, radiologic, and endoscopic studies, and, for patients with chest pain, cardiac studies have failed to clarify the cause for symptoms; and (b) when there is evidence of impaired function despite adequate reassurance. Patients to be tested must also have no contraindication to the administration of a drug with cholinergic properties. Based on available efficacy and safety data (7,8), intravenous edrophonium chloride (Tensilon, Roche Laboratories, Nutley, New Jersey) is the drug of choice for provocative testing.

1. After routine manometry, reposition the catheter assembly as described in Chapter 4.
2. Insert a No. 21 gauge scalp vein needle (E-Z 21 infusion set, Deseret Pharmaceutical Co., Inc., Sandy, Utah) into an accessible vein on the upper extremity. Flush tubing with sterile saline.

3. Check to see that atropine is on hand to reverse untoward effects from edrophonium administration.
4. Administer randomly either placebo (1 ml sterile saline fluid) or edrophonium (80 mcg/kg; 10 mg maximal dose) as a rapid intravenous injection.
5. Perform ten wet swallows over a 5-min period and record patient symptoms on tracing.
6. Repeat step 4 using the alternate agent, placebo or edrophonium, as an intravenous bolus.
7. Repeat step 5 by performing ten wet swallows over 5 min and recording patient symptoms on tracing.
8. Interpretation. A positive test occurs when injection of edrophonium, but not placebo, elicits the patient's chest pain *and* a manometric abnormality not observed on baseline testing.

Remove Catheter

Remove the catheter to conclude the study or leave it in place for pH probe testing (Chapter 6), potential difference measurement (Chapter 5), or Bernstein testing (Chapter 7).

Postprocedure

Patient may resume normal activities.

Complications

None reported with routine manometry. For provocative testing with edrophonium, drug side effects reported include dizziness, nausea, and abdominal cramps.

Interpretation

Figure 2 shows a schematic representation of the motility pattern elicited by swallows in a healthy subject.

Esophageal Manometric Data

Esophageal manometric data obtained in "normal subjects" (25) at North Carolina School of Medicine. 14 female, 11 male, ages 21 to 36, mean age 26. No history of systemic disease, GI disorders, medication, heartburn, dysphagia, chest pain, or odynophagia.

Instruments Used

Perfused-catheter system (1.1 mm ID), three catheters with lateral sensing orifices 5 cm apart, perfusion rate 0.6 ml/min. External transducers (Hewlett Packard Co. 1280C). Recorder/ Amplifier (Sanborn 7700 series), paper speed 1 mm/sec. Pneumohydraulic capillary infusion system (Arndorfer Medical Specialties Company, Greendale, Wisconsin). Belt pneumograph for swallows. Recording period 16 min with distal channel recording LES, middle and proximal channels 5 and 10 cm above LES in body, respectively.

Standard Data (Means ± SD)

Lower esophageal sphincter
1. LESP—mean 19.2 ± 6.9 mm Hg; range 9 to 32 mm Hg with peak = 11 to 40 mm Hg.
2. % LES relaxation (wet swallows)—mean 96 ± 10%; range of means 67 to 100%.

Esophageal body: primary peristalsis
1. Mean amplitude (wet swallows):
   a. Proximal channel—71 ± 26 mm Hg.
   b. Middle channel—65 ± 19 mm Hg.
2. Range of mean amplitudes (wet swallows):
   a. Proximal channel—35 to 120 mm Hg.
   b. Middle channel—27 to 100 mm Hg.
3. Mean duration (wet swallows):
   a. Proximal channel—4.8 ± 0.9 sec.
   b. Middle channel—4.8 ± 1.0 sec.
4. Range of mean duration (wet swallows):
   a. Proximal channel—3.3 to 6.2 sec.
   b. Middle channel—3.3 to 6.6 sec.
5. Propulsive versus nonpropulsive (simultaneous) contractions—94.5% propulsive and 5.5% nonpropulsive with wet swallows.

Esophageal body: primary peristalsis

1. Mean amplitude (dry swallows):

    a. Proximal channel—45 ± 21 mm Hg.

    b. Middle channel—46 ± 13 mm Hg.

2. Range of mean amplitudes (dry swallows):

    a. Proximal channel—21 to 112 mm Hg.

    b. Middle channel—25 to 81 mm Hg.

3. Mean duration (dry swallows):

    a. Proximal channel—4.7 ± 0.9 sec.

    b. Middle channel—4.8 ± 0.8 sec.

4. Range of mean duration (dry swallows):

    a. Proximal channel—2.8 to 6.3 sec.

    b. Middle channel—3.4 to 6.3 sec.

5. Propulsive vs nonpropulsive (simultaneous)—84% propulsive and 16% nonpropulsive with dry swallows.

Esophageal body: tertiary contractions

1. Present in 22/25 or 88% of subjects.

2. Proximal channel—number of tertiary waves ranged 0 to 52 in 16-min recording.

3. Middle channel—number of tertiary waves ranged 0 to 64 in 16-min recording.

4. Tertiary contractions were "infrequent" in 18/25 or 72%—i.e., <1 tertiary wave per minute.

5. Tertiary contractions were "frequent" in 7/25 or 28%—i.e., >1 tertiary wave per minute.

    a. Range of frequency was 16 to 116 waves/16 min.

    b. Runs of 2 and 3 waves common; runs of 6 and 8 waves seen in two different subjects; no symptoms in any subject.

6. Mean amplitude:

    a. Proximal channel—12 ± 3 mm Hg.

    b. Middle channel—12 ± 3 mm Hg.

7. Mean duration:

    a. Proximal channel—3.1 ± 0.5 sec.

    b. Middle channel—2.9 ± 0.4 sec.

Note. Amplitude of tertiary contractions significantly lower

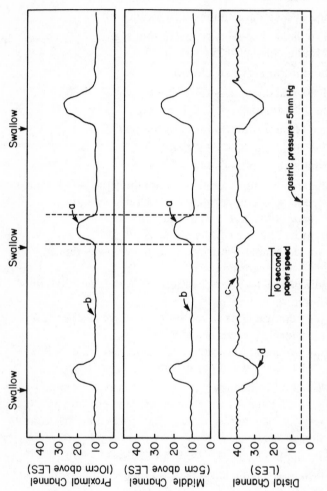

FIG. 3. Achalasia. Characteristic findings on manometry include (a) low-amplitude aperistaltic contractions with *all* swallows; (b) high resting pressure in the esophageal body; (c) high LES pressure; and (d) incomplete LES relaxation. For technical reasons, LES relaxation may appear complete on manometry in some subjects (1,10,11).

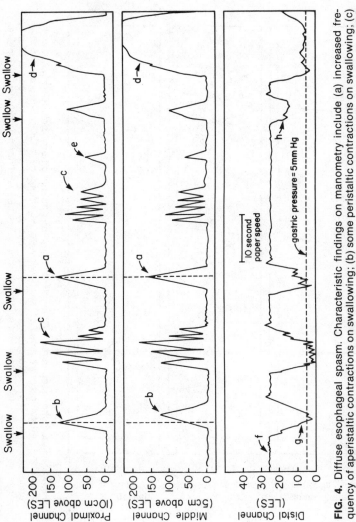

FIG. 4. Diffuse esophageal spasm. Characteristic findings on manometry include (a) increased frequency of aperistaltic contractions on swallowing; (b) some peristaltic contractions on swallowing; (c) repetitive contractions on swallowing; (d) high-amplitude long-duration contractions; and (e) tertiary waves. The LES may have (f) normal pressure; high pressure (not shown); (g) complete relaxation on swallowing; or (h) incomplete relaxation on swallowing (1,10).

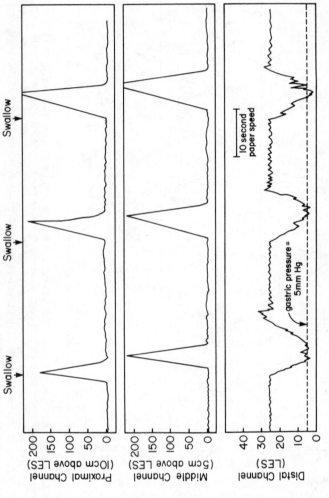

FIG. 5. "Nutcracker esophagus." Characteristic findings on manometry include frequent high-amplitude peristaltic contractions on swallowing (mean amplitude >120 mm Hg and/or peak amplitude of a single contraction >200 mm Hg). The duration of such contractions is usually prolonged, but this is not essential for the diagnosis. The LES is of normal pressure and relaxes completely on swallowing (1,10).

than amplitude of primary peristaltic waves and duration of tertiary contractions significantly shorter than primary peristaltic waves.

Figures 3 to 5 illustrate schematically some characteristic motor patterns in patients with symptomatic esophageal motor disease.

For provocative testing, see page 36.

REFERENCES

1. Cohen S (1979): Motor disorders of the esophagus. *N Engl J Med* 301:44–52.
2. Stef JJ, Dodds WJ, Hogan WJ, Linehan JH (1974): Esophageal manometry. Component analysis of systems used to record intraluminal pressure. *Proceedings of the Fourth International Symposium on Gastrointestinal Motility,* pp 337–346, Banff, Alberta, Canada.
3. Stef JJ, Dodds WJ, Hogan WJ, Linehan JH, Stewart ET (1974): Intraluminal esophageal manometry: an analysis of variables affecting recording fidelity of peristaltic pressures. *Gastroenterology* 67:221–230.
4. Arndorfer RC, Stef JJ, Dodds WJ, Linehan JH, Hogan WJ (1977): Improved infusion system for intraluminal esophageal manometry. *Gastroenterology* 73:23–37.
5. Hurwitz AL, Duranceau A, Haddad JK (1979): Esophageal manometric technique; and the performance of the esophageal motility study. In: *Disorders of Esophageal Motility,* edited by LH Smith Jr, pp 27–51. WB Saunders Co, Philadelphia.
6. Dodds WJ, Hogan WJ, Stef JJ, Miller WN, Lydon AB, Arndorfer RC (1975): A rapid pull-through technique for measuring lower esophageal sphincter pressure. *Gastroenterology* 68:437–443.
7. Richter JE, Hackshaw BT, Wu WC, Castell DO (1985): Edrophonium: a useful provocative test for esophageal chest pain. *Ann Intern Med* 103:14–21.
8. Benjamin SB, Richter JE, Cordova CM, Knuff TE, Castell DO (1983): Prospective manometric evaluation with pharmacologic provocation of patients with suspected esophageal motility dysfunction. *Gastroenterology* 84:893–901.
9. Benjamin SB, Gerhardt DC, Castell DO (1979): High amplitude, peristaltic esophageal contractions associated with chest pain and/or dysphagia. *Gastroenterology* 77:478–483.
10. Vantrappen G, Hellemans J (1982): Esophageal motor disorders.

In: *Diseases of the Esophagus,* edited by S Cohen, RD Soloway, pp 161–179. Churchill Livingstone, New York.

11. Katz PO, Richter JE, Cowan R, Castell DO (1986): Apparent complete lower esophageal sphincter relaxation in achalasia. *Gastroenterology* 90:978–983.

5 / Esophageal Potential Difference Measurements

Roy C. Orlando

The esophageal transmural electrical potential difference (PD) in humans and rabbits is generated by the combination of active electrolyte (primarily Na^+) transport from lumen to blood and epithelial resistance to passive electrolyte movements in either direction (1,2). The PD (or voltage) is therefore a marker of epithelial function and integrity, and one that can be recorded *in vivo*. The normal *in vivo* esophageal PD in humans is approximately -15 ± 5 mV (mean $\pm$ 1 SD) (3,4). When the esophageal epithelium is altered by disease, the PD frequently becomes abnormal, and the type of abnormality in PD (i.e., too high or too low) may suggest the type and extent of disease (4–7). Although the measurement of PD is still experimental, the simplicity of its measurement by the perfused catheter technique (3) and the success of our studies (4,5) prompted its inclusion here.

Indications

1. To screen for esophageal mucosal disease in patients with dysphagia, heartburn, and/or chest pain.
2. As an aid to the diagnosis of Barrett's esophagus.

Contraindications

1. Poor patient cooperation.
2. Patients with cardiac instability or other conditions where vagal stimulation is poorly tolerated.

Preparation

1. Nothing by mouth within 6 to 8 hr of study.
2. Obtain informed, written consent.

Equipment

For setup, see Fig. 1.

1. Harvard pump with plastic syringe.
2. Pressure transducer (Model No. 1280-C, Hewlett Packard Co., Palo Alto, California).
3. Agar bridges—polyethylene tubing (PE 280) filled with 4% agar-lactated Ringer's solution.
4. Standard manometric catheter assembly (polyvinyl catheter, 1.1 mm internal diameter with 1 mm lateral sensing orifice).
5. Pen Recorder (Hewlett Packard eight-channel recorder, model 7758 A) with a paper speed 1 mm/sec. Only two recorder channels, one for pressure and one for PD, are required for this study.

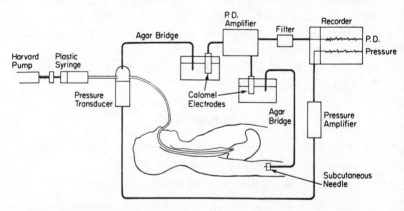

FIG. 1. Schematic representation of a perfused catheter method for obtaining simultaneous esophageal pressure PD measurements. *Note:* The standard manometric catheter is converted into a PD sensor by perfusing with lactated Ringer's solution instead of water, and the same orifice is used to sense both PD and pressure. The beakers in which the calomel electrodes are placed contain a saturated solution of KCl.

6. Reference electrode: lactated Ringer agar-filled No. 19 gauge scalp vein needle and tubing (E-Z 19 infusion set, Deseret Pharmaceutical Co., Inc., Sandy, Utah).
7. KCl solution (saturated).
8. Calomel reference electrodes (Fisher Scientific Co., Pittsburgh, Pennsylvania).
9. Bioelectric amplifier (high impedance—10^{12} ohms, electrically isolated) (Electronics Dept., University of North Carolina School of Medicine, Chapel Hill, North Carolina).
10. Filter—battery-operated band reject with 40-db attenuation factor (Electronics Dept., University of North Carolina School of Medicine, Chapel Hill, North Carolina).

Procedure[1]

1. Pass a standard manometric catheter assembly through the nose into midesophagus and flush the distal esophagus with 30 cc Ringer's lactate.
2. Advance the assembly until the distal channel records gastric pressure (for details, see Chapter 4). *Note*. The catheter for the distal channel should be connected to the pressure transducer with a modified dome. This dome, which is fitted with a lactated Ringer agar bridge, enables the same catheter to serve as a PD probe.
3. Disconnect the modified pressure transducer from the Arndorfer pump used for manometry and connect it to a Harvard pump (Fig. 1). The plastic syringe in the Harvard pump should be filled with Ringer's solution and perfused at a rate of 1.9 ml/min.
4. Insert the scalp vein needle (agar-filled No. 19 butterfly) into the subcutaneous tissue on the volar surface of the forearm. Place the free end of the agar-filled tubing from the butterfly into one beaker with KCl. This beaker also has a calomel electrode that is connected to one terminal of the bioelectric amplifier.

---

[1] For more detailed account, see ref. 3.

5. Place the free end of the agar bridge connected to the modified pressure transducer into a second beaker of KC1. The calomel electrode from this second beaker is connected to the second terminal of the bioelectric amplifier (Fig. 1).

6. Calibration:

   a. Determine offset potential between calomel electrodes by placing both in same beaker of KC1. If voltage ≥ 2 mV, replace electrodes before study.

   b. Set the zero baseline by recording PD with the apparatus connected as shown in Fig. 1 but short circuited with another lactated Ringer agar bridge connecting the two solutions of KC1.

   c. Disconnect the calomel leads from the amplifier and insert leads from an independent voltage source. Input 20 to 50 mV and check to see if an appropriate deflection is recorded on the tracing. *Note.* Our recorder has two settings, 5 and 10 mV per box; the latter is used for all clinical studies.

   d. Reconnect the apparatus as shown in Fig. 1 and proceed with a station pull-through as described below at a paper speed of 1 mm/sec.

7. The station pull-through is performed by gradually withdrawing the catheter assembly at 1-cm increments every 5 sec from stomach to upper esophagus. Advance catheter assembly back into stomach and repeat pull-through two more times to ensure reproducibility.

8. Troubleshooting: Technically poor recordings are usually the result of:

   a. Inadequate Ringer's solution perfusing the esophagus (empty syringe, faulty pump)

   b. Poor contact of agar bridge with Ringer's solution in dome of pressure transducer or with subcutaneous interstitial fluid (avoid air bubbles, reposition and/or replace needle)

   c. Defective agar bridges (air bubbles or broken agar column)

   d. Short circuiting of PD by electrolytes spilled on transducer (clean dome of transducer with deionized water).

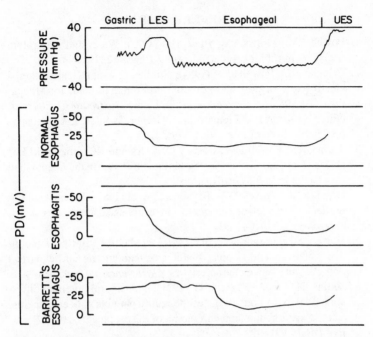

FIG. 2. Schematic representation of pressure–PD profiles obtained on station pull-through from stomach to upper esophageal sphincter (UES). Three different esophageal conditions are illustrated: normal, esophagitis, and Barrett's. Since the PD and pressure-sensing orifice are the same, the pressure profile identifies the location of the recorded PD. In the normal esophagus, the transition from the more negative gastric PD to the esophageal PD occurs within the LES. The normal esophageal PD remains between −5 mV and −25 mV. In esophagitis, the PD approaches zero at the area of damage. With Barrett's esophagus (columnar epithelium), the PD approximates that of the gastric PD (−25 mV).

Postprocedure

Patient may resume normal activities.

Complications

None reported.

Interpretation

See Fig. 2.

REFERENCES

1. Powell DW, Morris SM, Boyd DD (1975): Water and electrolyte transport in rabbit esophagus. *Am J Physiol* 229:438–443.
2. Orlando RC, Powell DW (1984): Studies of esophageal epithelial electrolyte transport and potential difference in man. In: *Mechanisms of Mucosal Protection in the Upper Gastrointestinal Tract,* edited by A Allen, G Flemstrom, A Garner, W Silen, LA Turnberg, pp 75–79. Raven Press, New York.
3. Turner KS, Powell DW, Carney CN, Orlando RC, Bozymski EM (1978): Transmural electrical potential difference in the mammalian esophagus in vivo. *Gastroenterology* 75:286–291.
4. Orlando RC, Powell DW, Bryson JC, et al (1982): Esophageal potential difference measurements in esophageal disease. *Gastroenterology* 83:1026–1032.
5. Herlihy KJ, Orlando RC, Bryson JC, et al (1984): Barrett's esophagus: clinical, endoscopic, histologic, manometric and electrical potential difference characteristics. *Gastroenterology* 86:436–444.
6. Vidins EI, Fox JAE, Beck IT (1971): Transmural potential difference (PD) in the body of the esophagus in patients with esophagitis, Barrett's epithelium and carcinoma of the esophagus. *Am J Digestive Dis* 16:991–999.
7. Khamis B, Kennedy C, Finucane J, Doyle S (1978): Transmural potential difference: diagnostic value in gastro-esophageal reflux. *Gut* 19:396–398.

6 / pH Probe for Reflux (Tuttle Test)

Roy C. Orlando

The Tuttle test fills the need for a simple sensitive method of documenting gastroesophageal reflux (1–3). Since intra-esophageal pH (pH $\geq$ 6) is normally higher than that of the stomach (pH 1–3), a pH probe positioned within the esophagus will record a fall in pH when gastroesophageal reflux occurs. Although reflux also can be demonstrated by barium contrast study of the upper gastrointestinal tract and gastrointestinal scintiscanning (4), the former test is moderately insensitive (3), and the latter requires more elaborate equipment than the Tuttle test.

Indications

1. Patients in whom there is a need to document objectively gastroesophageal reflux (e.g., those with atypical chest pain or aspiration pneumonia).
2. Patients in whom serial measurements would help establish the efficacy of medical and/or surgical antireflux therapy.

Contraindications

1. Poor patient cooperation.
2. Patients with cardiac instability or other conditions where vagal stimulation is poorly tolerated.
3. Active peptic ulcer disease.

Preparation

1. Give nothing by mouth for $\geq$8 hr.
2. Obtain informed, written consent.

Equipment

1. pH electrode (MI-506 Microelectrodes, Inc., London-derry, New Hampshire). Alternative: Beckman 39042 Glass Electrode (Beckman Instruments, Inc., Fullerton, California).
2. Reference electrode (EKG electrode and paste).
3. Esophageal manometric equipment (see Chapter 4, Esophageal Manometry).
4. 0.1 N HCl.
5. Standard pH test solutions.
6. Battery-powered pH meter (Beckman Laboratory model, Beckman Instruments, Fullerton, California) or pH meter with electrically isolated circuit for patient safety.

Procedure and Interpretation

1. The pH probe and reference electrode are attached to the pH meter and calibrated with standard pH solutions of 1, 4, and 7 as illustrated in Fig. 1A.
2. Following calibration, firmly tape the pH probe to a standard manometric catheter so that the pH recording tip extends 1 to 2 cm proximal to the end of the catheter. *Note.* The MI-506 Flexible pH electrode is small enough (outer diameter 1.3 mm) to be passed through some manometry assemblies made with a central large-bore catheter (Arndorfer Medical Specialties Company, Greendale, Wisconsin).
3. Connect the manometric equipment as previously described (Chapter 4) and pass the entire assembly into the stomach (Fig. 1B).
4. With the patient now supine, check the stomach pH. It should be <4. If the pH is >4 and a recheck of the equipment indicates no malfunction, skip to the "acid-load test" (item 7, below). If the stomach pH is <4, pull the assembly into the esophagus so that the pH electrode is located 5 cm above the manometrically localized lower esophageal sphincter (LES).
5. Tape the assembly to the nose and check the intraesophageal pH. If the pH is still at the level recorded in the stom-

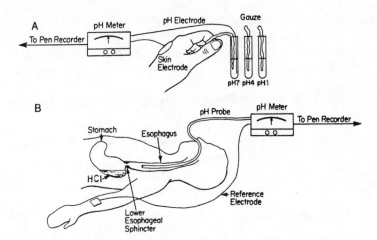

FIG. 1. A: Method for *in vivo* calibration of pH probe. **B:** Schematic representation of the setup used for the pH probe (Tuttle) test for reflux. *Note:* Maneuvers such as Valsalva, Müller, straight-leg raising, and abdominal compression are performed before and, if negative for reflux, after acid loading (300 cc 0.1 N HCl placed in stomach). The pH probe extends just distal to the manometric catheter and is located 5 cm above the LES.

ach, ask the patient to swallow until the pH ≥6. *Note.* If frequent swallows fail to raise the pH to >4, the patient has free reflux.

6. If free reflux is not observed (i.e., pH in the esophagus maintained ≥6), the patient performs two Valsalva, Müller, and straight-leg-raising maneuvers, followed by two manual abdominal compressions in the supine position. A drop in esophageal pH to <4 during or shortly after any two maneuvers is considered a positive test for reflux. If belching or burping occurs, maneuvers should be interrupted and the results not counted. This is because belching or burping lowers LES pressure and thereby produces a false-positive test for reflux.

7. Acid-load test. If no reflux is demonstrated during basal testing, the following acid-load test is performed: Advance the entire assembly into the stomach and infuse 300 cc 0.1 N HCl through the polyvinyl catheters. Withdraw the assembly into the esophagus and again fix the pH electrode in place 5 cm above the LES. With the esophageal pH

restored to pH ⩾6, repeat the maneuvers described in item 6 (above). A fall in esophageal pH to <4 for any two maneuvers after acid loading is also considered a positive test.
8. This concludes the test and the assembly can be removed.

Postprocedure

1. Patient may resume normal activities.
2. If acid loading has been performed, we usually give 30 cc antacid after the procedure.

Complications

None reported.

REFERENCES

1. Tuttle SG, BeHarello A, Grossman MI (1960): Esophageal acid perfusion test and a gastroesophageal reflux test in patients with esophagitis. *Gastroenterology* 38:861–872.
2. Benz LJ, Hootkin LA, Margulies S, Donner MW, Cauthorne RT, Hendrix TR (1972): A comparison of clinical measurements of gastroesophageal reflux. *Gastroenterology* 62:1–5.
3. Bombeck CT, Helfrich GB, Nuhus LM (1970): Planning surgery for reflux esophagitis and hiatal hernia. *Surg Clin North Am* 50:29–44.
4. Fisher RS, Malmud LS, Roberts GS, Lobis IF (1976): Gastroesophageal (GE) scintiscanning to detect and quantitate GE reflux. *Gastroenterology* 70:301–307.

7 / Bernstein (Acid Perfusion) Test

Robert S. Sandler

The Bernstein test is a clinical procedure used to determine if a patient's symptoms are due to acid reflux. The test was devised to distinguish between angina pectoris and esophageal pain in the patient with atypical chest pain (1). It has been shown to correlate with esophagitis symptoms but not with the severity of esophagitis (2). The test is not specific, since patients with gastritis may also have a positive test (3), and there may be false negatives. While the study is simple to perform, it may be difficult to interpret, since it relies on subjective responses by the patient (4).

The mechanism of pain production is uncertain but may be due to direct stimulation of exposed esophageal sensory receptors (2). Recent analysis of esophageal sensitivity in patients with esophagitis suggests that pH is not the sole factor responsible for heartburn (5).

The procedure appears to be quite safe. Acid perfusion does not produce gross esophagoscopic abnormalities. The test does not produce angina or gastrointestinal bleeding. In patients with coronary artery disease, a positive Bernstein test may produce ST segment depression on EKG consistent with myocardial ischemia (6).

Indication

To determine if the patient's symptoms are esophageal in origin. The test evaluates symptoms alone and does not indicate the presence of esophagitis or acid reflux.

Contraindication

Active or recent bleeding from a peptic process.

Preparation of Patient

The patient should be fasting.

Equipment

1. Nasogastric tube (14–16 French). If the patient has undergone esophageal manometry, the manometry catheter may be used.
2. Three-way stopcock.
3. Reservoirs of normal saline solution and 0.1 N HCl.
4. Lubricant.

Procedure

1. Place the patient in an upright position.
2. Pass the lubricated nasogastric tube (see Chapter 1, Gastrointestinal Intubation) so that the perfusing tip is 30 to 35 cm from the nares.
3. Connect the nasogastric (NG) tube to the reservoirs of 0.1 N HCl and normal saline solution via the three-way stopcock. Place the reservoirs behind the patient so that the flow can be switched without the patient's knowledge (Fig. 1).
4. Instruct the patient to indicate whether the drip produces typical symptoms or some new complaint.
5. Drip normal saline solution at 100 to 120 drops per minute for 5 min.
6. After 5 min, switch the flow to 0.1 N HCl using the three-way stopcock.
7. Allow the acid to flow until symptoms appear or until 30 min have elapsed. Disregard transient or momentary symptoms. Symptoms in a positive test are persistent and usually progressive in severity as long as administration of acid continues.
8. If symptoms appear, switch back to normal saline solution. The symptoms may decrease in 3 or 4 min. If the symptoms disappear with saline infusion, switch the flow back to 0.1 N HCl. The symptoms will reappear if they are due to esophageal sensitivity.

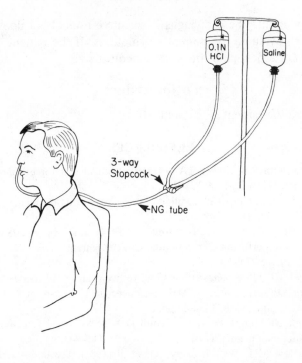

FIG. 1. Bernstein test. Solutions of 0.1 N HCl and saline solution are placed behind the patient. The flow can be switched by turning the three-way stopcock without the patient's knowledge.

9. Record whether acid perfusion reproduces the patient's typical symptoms, results in heartburn, or produces a new sensation. All of these types of pain indicate a positive Bernstein test but have different implications. Confusion might result if the test is simply reported as positive without a description of the symptoms.

Interpretation

If the patient's symptoms are reproduced, the test provides evidence for the esophageal origin of the complaints. Saline infusion may not relieve the symptoms in all patients and should not be a required criterion for a positive test (7). If the patient complains of burning discomfort (heartburn), the study indicates that the esophagus is sensitive to acid but does not help to evaluate the patient's symptoms. If the patient complains of a new pain, the test is inconclusive.

Postprocedure

Give the patient 30 cc antacid.

REFERENCES

1. Bernstein LM, Baker TA (1958): A clinical test for esophagitis. *Gastroenterology* 34:760–781.
2. Dodds WJ, Hogan WJ, Miller WM (1976): Reflux esophagitis. *Am J Digestive Dis* 21:49–67.
3. DeMorges-Filho JPP, Bettarello A (1974): Lack of specificity of the acid perfusion test in duodenal ulcer patients. *Am J Digestive Dis* 19:785–790.
4. Pope CE (1983): Gastrointestinal reflux disease. In: *Gastrointestinal Disease,* edited by MH Sleisenger, JS Fordtran, pp 449–476. WB Saunders Co, Philadelphia.
5. Price SF, Smithson KW, Castell DO (1978): Food sensitivity in reflux esophagitis. *Gastroenterology* 75:240–243.
6. Mellow MH, Walt L, Haye O, et al (1981): Cardiovascular response to esophageal acid perfusion in coronary disease. *Gastroenterology* 80:1230.
7. Winnan GR, Meyer CT, McCallum RW (1982): Interpretation of the Bernstein test: a reappraisal of criteria. *Ann Intern Med* 96:320–322.

8 / Gastric Secretory Testing

Kenneth B. Klein

Gastric secretory testing assesses the basal and maximal capacity of the stomach to produce acid. Because of a number of important diagnostic and therapeutic advances over the past decade, gastric secretory testing now has rather limited clinical usefulness.

Indications

Helpful in Some Circumstances

1. In recurrent peptic ulcer disease, especially after ulcer surgery:
   a. To rule out hypersecretory states (e.g., Zollinger-Ellison syndrome, retained antrum);
   b. To test for completeness of vagotomy.
2. To determine the optimal dosage of acid-lowering drugs in Zollinger-Ellison syndrome.
3. To evaluate the patient with hypergastrinemia:
   a. Is it "pathological" (e.g., Zollinger-Ellison syndrome, G-cell hyperplasia)?
   b. Is it a physiological response to hypochlorhydria (e.g., atrophic gastritis)?

Rarely Helpful

1. To establish the diagnosis of Zollinger-Ellison Syndrome. Serum gastrin levels and gastrin response to secretin infusion have greater sensitivity and specificity than measurement of

acid secretion, even with determination of the basal acid output/maximal acid output (BAO/MAO) ratio (1,2).

2. To diagnose pernicious anemia. Serum B_{12} levels and the Schilling test are more specific; most cases of achlorhydria are not associated with pernicious anemia.

3. To predict the likelihood of ulcer recurrence after surgery. Measurement of either preoperative or postoperative acid secretion is in general not useful (3).

Virtually Never Helpful

1. For the evaluation of nonulcer (or "X-ray negative") dyspepsia.
2. In the routine evaluation of patients with peptic ulcer disease.
3. To help determine the optimal type of ulcer surgery.
4. To distinguish benign from malignant gastric ulcers. Only 20% of gastric cancers occur in the setting of achlorhydria (4). Further, benign ulcers occasionally occur in stomachs that produce little or no acid.

Contraindications

1. Gastric outlet obstruction.
2. Recent upper gastrointestinal bleeding.
3. Potential obstruction to free passage of a nasogastric tube, such as prior nasopharyngeal surgery, Zenker's diverticulum, or high-grade esophageal stricture.
4. Recent upper respiratory infection or allergic rhinitis.

Preparation

1. Discontinue all medications that might affect gastric secretion at least 24 hr prior to testing. Such drugs include H_2 blockers, antihistamines, cholinergics, anticholinergics, tranquilizers, antidepressants, and carbonic anhydrase inhibitors. If the patient is experiencing peptic ulcer pain, antacids may be used for symptomatic relief during this period.

2. Nothing by mouth after midnight.
3. Explain the nature of the procedure to the patient in detail.

Equipment

1. A 14 to 18 French nasogastric tube. A double-lumen (vented) tube is preferred.
2. Supplies for passing the tube (see Chapter 1).
3. A 50- or 60-ml "catheter-tip" syringe.
4. Pentagastrin, 6 μg/kg.
5. Intermittent suction pump (desirable, but not essential).
6. Eight 120-cc gastric fluid collection containers.
7. Acid-titrating equipment, including a pH meter, graduated burette, small beakers, and 0.1 N NaOH.

Procedure

1. Introduce the nasogastric (NG) tube into the nose and advance it until the tip lies in the stomach (see Chapter 1).
2. Aspirate stomach contents. If food particles or more than a few hundred milliliters of fluid are present, the test should not be done, and the reason for this finding determined (e.g., the patient ate breakfast, gastric outlet obstruction, motility disorder).
3. Position the tip of the tube in the most dependent portion of the stomach. This may be determined by fluoroscopy or equally well by the "water-recovery test" (5,6). In this test, 20 to 50 ml water is introduced into the stomach via the NG tube or by asking the patient to swallow it. Then, as much of the water as possible is aspirated through the tube using the catheter-tip syringe. If recovery is greater than 90%, placement is adequate.
4. Collect gastric juice either by machine suction (preferably intermittent) or by frequent manual aspiration. Ensure tube patency by injecting small quantities of air every 5 min or so. Note the presence of blood or bile, either of which may result in erroneously low acid values.
5. For routine gastric analysis, it is not necessary to prevent the swallowing of sputum (e.g., by use of a dental sucker) or to use a marker to correct for gastric fluid loss through

the pylorus. The patient may sit comfortably in a chair; precise positioning is not important (5).

6. *BAO collection*. Collect gastric secretions for the first hour in four 15-min samples.

7. *Pentagastrin injection*. After the first hour, inject pentagastrin, 6 μg/kg subcutaneously, which will maximally stimulate acid production (7). Warn the patient of these possible side effects: flushing, nausea, abdominal pain, dizziness, palpitations, and faintness (usually they are mild and transient).

8. *Peak acid output (PAO) collection*. During the postinjection hour, again collect gastric secretions in four 15-min samples.

9. Calculate basal and peak acid outputs (see below).

Postprocedure

1. Repeat the water-recovery test to document that final tube placement was appropriate.

2. Aspirate any remaining gastric fluid.

3. Remove the NG tube.

4. Resume medications.

Interpretation: Measurement of Acid Content and Calculation of BAO and PAO

1. Measure and record the volume of each of the eight 15-min collections. (*Note.* Figure 1 is an example of a worksheet that we find useful in the recording and calculation of gastric secretory testing data.)

2. If particulate matter is present, centrifuge the sample.

3. An aliquot (e.g., 5 ml) from each of the eight collections is then titrated with 0.1 N NaOH to pH 7.0.

4. Calculate the acid content of each 15-min collection as follows:

   a. (ml NaOH needed for titration to pH 7) $\times$ 0.1 = mEq H^+ in aliquot

   b. mEq H^+ in 15-min collection

   $$= \frac{\text{volume of collection}}{\text{volume of aliquot}} \times \text{mEq } H^+ \text{ in aliquot}$$

Patient Name: _____

Weight: _____ kg

Indication: _____

Patient #: _____

Date: ___ ___ ___
       M   D   Y

I. FIRST HOUR - BAO

Sample No.	Scheduled Time (mins)	Actual Clock Time (0-2400) Start	Actual Clock Time (0-2400) End	Appearance	(a) Vol (mls)	(b) pH	(c) ml 0.1 N NaOH to pH 7.0 (5 ml aliquot)	(d) meq H⁺/ml Sample (c ÷ 50)	(e) meq H⁺/Total Sample (a x d)
1	0 - 15								
2	15 - 30								
3	30 - 45								
4	45 - 60								

BAO = Σe = _____ meq H⁺/hr

II. SECOND HOUR - PAO and MAO

Pentagastrin injection (6 μg/kg): _____ μg (_____ ml)   Time of injection: _____ (0-2400)

Sample No.	Scheduled Time (mins)	Actual Clock Time (0-2400) Start	Actual Clock Time (0-2400) End	Appearance	(a) Vol (mls)	(b) pH	(c) ml 0.1 N NaOH to pH 7.0 (5 ml aliquot)	(d) meq H⁺/ml Sample (c ÷ 50)	(e) meq H⁺/Total Sample (a x d)
5	0 - 15								
6	15 - 30								
7	30 - 45								
8	45 - 60								

PAO = Two highest adjacent (e) column values x 2 = _____ meq H⁺/hr

MAO = Σe = _____ meq H⁺/hr

_____
Signature

FIG. 1. Gastric secretory testing worksheet.

TABLE 1. Gastric Secretory Testing: Typical Values

	BAO (mEq H^+/hr)		MAO (mEq H^+/hr)		PAO (mEq H^+/hr)	
	Average	Range	Average	Range	Average	Range
Normal subjects						
Males	2.5	0–10	25	7–50	35	10–60
Females	1.5	0–6	15	5–30	25	8–40
Duodenal ulcer						
Males	5.0	0.1–15	40	15–60	45	15–70
Females	3.0	0.1–15	30	10–45	35	15–55
Gastric ulcer						
Males	1.5	0–8	20	5–40		
Females	1.0	0–5	12	3–25		
Zollinger-Ellison syndrome, both sexes	40	10–90	65	30–120		

5. BAO, expressed as mEq H^+/hr, is the sum of the acid content of the four 15-min collections made during the first hour.

6. PAO, expressed as mEq H^+/hr, is determined by adding the acid content of the two adjacent 15-min postpentagastrin collections with the highest values, then multiplying by 2. PAO represents the greatest acid output of which the parietal cell mass is capable. It is also the most reproducible of the various measures of acid stimulation (7).

7. MAO, expressed as mEq H^+/hr, has been defined in various ways but is generally taken to represent the sum of the acid content of the four 15-min collections following pentagastrin administration.

8. See Table 1 for representative values.

REFERENCES

1. Malagelada JR, Davis CS, O'Fallon WM, Go VLW (1982): Laboratory diagnosis of gastrinoma: I. a prospective evaluation of gastric analysis and fasting serum gastrin levels. *Mayo Clin Proc* 57:211–218.

2. Malagelada JR, Glanzman SC, Go VLW (1982): Laboratory diagnosis of gastrinoma: II. a prospective study of gastrin challenge tests. *Mayo Clin Proc* 57:219–226.

3. Johnston D, Pickford IR, Walker BE, Goligher JC (1975): Highly selective vagotomy for duodenal ulcer: do hypersecretors need antrectomy? *Br Med J* 1:716–718.
4. Baron JH (1979): Gastric ulcer and carcinoma. In: *Clinical Tests of Gastric Secretion: History, Methodology, and Interpretation,* pp 86–97. Oxford University Press, New York.
5. Hassan MA, Hobsley M (1970): Positioning of subject and of nasogastric tube during a gastric secretory study. *Br Med J* 1:458–460.
6. Findlay JM, Prescott RJ, Sircus W (1972): Comparative evaluation of water recovery test and fluoroscopic screening in positioning a nasogastric tube during gastric secretory studies. *Br Med J* 4:458–461.
7. Baron JH (1979): Maximal stimuli. In: *Clinical Tests of Gastric Secretion: History, Methodology, and Interpretation,* pp 25–35. Oxford University Press, New York.

9 / Secretin Test

Roy C. Orlando

The pancreas, by virtue of its location, has been a difficult organ to study. Nonetheless, for over 30 years, the availability of the secretin test has helped diagnose chronic pancreatitis and pancreatic cancer in many patients (1–3). Since the advent of ultrasonography, computerized axial tomography, arteriography, and endoscopic retrograde cholangiopancreatography, reliance on the secretin test to diagnose these conditions has appropriately diminished. Yet the test remains important as a method for obtaining pancreatic cytologic specimens and documenting abnormalities in pancreatic exocrine function.

Indications

For evaluating patients with abdominal pain, weight loss, or steatorrhea in whom the diagnosis of chronic pancreatitis or pancreatic cancer is suspected.

Contraindications

1. Acute pancreatitis.
2. Uncooperative patient.
3. Allergy to secretin.

Preparation

1. Nothing by mouth after midnight.
2. Obtain informed, written consent.

Equipment

1. Dreiling tube (Davol Rubber Company): a double-lumen tube with one set of aspiration ports positioned to retrieve gastric contents and the other for duodenal contents.

2. Secretin-Kabi (Greenwich, Connecticut); same as secretin-GIH. Replaces secretin-Boots, which is a less pure formulation with greater potential for allergic reactions.
3. Collection bottles.
4. Basin with ice.
5. Two 50-cc catheter-tipped syringes for aspirating gastric and duodenal juice and one 10-cc syringe for administering secretin.
6. pH paper.
7. No. 21 gauge scalp vein needle and tubing.
8. Suction units: wall or portable.
9. Fluoroscopy unit.

Procedure

1. The Dreiling tube is passed by mouth into the stomach and then guided with the aid of fluoroscopy through the duodenum to the ligament of Treitz.
2. With the patient supine and the tube in proper position (Fig. 1), aspirate juice from the duodenal and gastric chan-

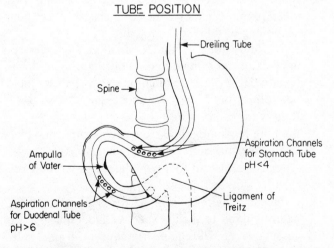

TUBE POSITION

FIG. 1. Schematic representation of a Dreiling tube properly positioned for performance of the secretin test. *Note.* All gastric aspiration ports are within the stomach, and all duodenal ports are distal to the pylorus such that they only aspirate duodenal contents.

nels using different 50-cc syringes. The duodenal juice should be alkaline and usually bile stained, whereas the gastric juice should be acidic (check with pH paper).

3. After verifying that the tube is properly positioned, tape it to the nose and aspirate gastric contents until there is no return.

4. Collection of baseline sample:

   a. Connect both gastric and duodenal channels to a suction unit for continuous low suctioning at 25 to 40 mm Hg for 10 to 20 min.

   b. Discard gastric juice.

   c. The duodenal juice collected is the basal sample.

   d. Measure its total volume; then handle the sample as described in item 6,f (below).

   e. Reinstitute suctioning of both gastric and duodenal secretions.

5. Administer secretin-Kabi 0.1 CU i.v. to test for allergy. If there is no reaction after 1 min, then administer the full dose of 1 CU/kg i.v. over 1 min.

6. Collection of stimulated samples:

   a. Immediately begin to collect the first of four consecutive 20-min samples (labeled in order) by continuous suctioning of duodenal contents.

   b. Measure the total volume for each sample before placing part of the sample into a collection tube for bicarbonate (HCO_3^-) determination. *Note.* Tubes should be kept on ice until ready for processing.

   c. Repeat for each sample.

   d. Pool the remaining fluid from each sample and place it in a beaker on ice for cytologic study.

   e. After collecting all four samples, remove the Dreiling tube by slow withdrawal.

   f. *Immediately* take the samples for cytology and HCO_3^- determination to their respective laboratories for processing. *Note.* The chemistry request slip *must* indicate that HCO_3^- determinations need to be carried out accurately; i.e., dilutions need to be made to obtain the final concentration of HCO_3^-. If this is not done,

TABLE 1. Secretin Test Results for Diagnosing Chronic Pancreatitis and Pancreatic Cancer

	Diagnosis	
	Chronic Pancreatitis	Pancreatic Cancer
Cytology	Negative	Positive (60% of cases)
HCO_3^-	<90 mEq/liter in all samples	≥90 mEq/liter in one or more samples
Total volume[a]	≥2 ml/kg	<2 ml/kg

[a] Sum of all sample volumes after secretin divided by weight in kilograms.

HCO_3^- will be reported as >40 mEq/liter, a level that has no diagnostic value.

Postprocedure

The patient may resume normal activities.

Interpretation

Although earlier versions of the secretin test included amylase assays, these have been omitted here because of their limited value in diagnosing chronic pancreatitis and pancreatic cancer.

Pitfalls Affecting Results

1. Inadequate aspiration of gastric contents can lead to acidification of the duodenal juice, producing falsely low HCO_3^-.
2. Inadequate collection of duodenal contents can lead to falsely low total volume.
3. Poor tube position can cause errors in HCO_3^- and/or volume.
4. Patients with prior vagotomy, inflammatory bowel disease, or currently on anticholinergic therapy may have low values in the absence of pancreatic pathology.
5. Except for a *positive* cytology, which is conclusive for cancer, the data obtained (i.e., volume and HCO_3^-) should be viewed as objective evidence in support of chronic pan-

creatitis or pancreatic cancer. However, since the patterns shown may overlap in approximately 5% of cases, these findings are not pathognomonic for these disorders.

Complications

Allergic reactions (secretin-Boots)—none reported with secretin-Kabi.

REFERENCES

1. Dreiling DA (1975): Pancreatic secretory testing. *Gut* 16:653–657.
2. Banks PA (1979): Diagnosis of chronic pancreatitis. In: *Pancreatitis,* edited by HM Spiro, pp 202–204. Plenum Medical Book Company, New York.
3. Brooks FP (1980): Chronic and chronic relapsing pancreatitis. In: *Diseases of the Exocrine Pancreas,* edited by LH Smith Jr, pp 51–54. WB Saunders, Philadelphia.

10 / Intubation for Small Bowel Biopsy and Duodenal Aspiration

William D. Heizer

Duodenal intubation of most patients requires less than 45 min and may be only mildly uncomfortable when correctly performed. The minimal risk and discomfort of jejunal biopsy allow for earlier and more frequent use on outpatients as well as hospitalized patients. Diagnostic biopsies may be indicated not only for diarrhea and weight loss but also for osteopenia, bone pain, anemia, fever, arthritis, serositis, and central nervous system dysfunction. Preparation and interpretation of histological slides from these specimens require special skill, and biopsies should not be attempted without a commitment to special handling by the pathology department.

Indications

Small Bowel Biopsy

To support, confirm, or exclude diseases of the small intestine (1,2). Several different devices are available for obtaining jejunal biopsies:

1. Multipurpose tube (Rubin-Quinton) (3) in one-hole, two-hole, and four-hole models. Because proximal small intestinal lesions may be patchy, the four-hole version is usually preferable for routine use.
2. One-hole steerable device (Medi-Tech) (4).
3. Carey capsule. This is often used for pediatric biopsies but is acceptable in adults. The specimen obtained is somewhat more broad and less deep than those obtained with the multipurpose instrument.

Duodenal Aspiration

1. To diagnose giardiasis.
2. To diagnose bacterial overgrowth.
3. To determine the presence of cholesterol crystals and white blood cells in patients with suspected gallbladder disease.
4. To collect pancreatic fluid as part of the secretin test.

The following discussion, except where indicated, pertains to small bowel biopsy with a Rubin-Quinton tube.

Contraindications

1. Uncooperative patient.
2. Uncorrectable coagulation disorder (see Chapter 22, contraindications, item 2).

Preparation

1. Read the instruction manual that comes with the multipurpose biopsy tube.
2. Test instrument for proper assembly and for air leaks:
   a. Assemble the tube.
   b. Pull the wire to close the ports and further occlude the ports between the thumb and forefinger.
   c. Immerse the assembled tube in water.
   d. Force air into the tube with syringe.
   e. If any air leaks are noted, these areas should be marked, dried, and repaired by rubbing a cotton-tipped applicator saturated with tetrahydrofuran lightly back and forth across the area including the hole. This dissolves some of the vinyl rubber and lets it flow into the hole.
3. Determine if there is a personal or family history of bleeding diathesis.
4. Determine the hematocrit, platelet count (or adequate on smear), PT, PTT, TCT (p. 149).
5. Have the patient sign consent form.
6. The patient's stomach should be empty.

7. Give topical anesthesia with cetacaine or lidocaine.
8. Very rarely, intravenous diazepam and/or meperidine are given.

Equipment

1. Rubin-Quinton multipurpose tube (or Medi-Tech steerable tube, Carey capsule).
2. Fluoroscope.
3. Mouth suction.
4. Patient's most recent upper gastrointestinal series.

Procedure

See Fig. 1.

1. Test the instrument to make sure the ports will open and close, even when the tube is coiled in a 6-in.-diameter circle. The pull wire protruding from the handle should be adjusted so that when the handle is pushed in as far as it will go, the capsule will open, but the amount of pressure exerted is not enough to damage the tube.
2. Tighten the Allen screw to hold the pull wire firmly in the chuck.
3. Pull the activator wire to close the ports of the capsule and slide the rubber O-ring down the shaft of the handle to prevent accidental opening of the ports.
4. Place the tip of the lubricated tube with the mercury bolus in the patient's pharynx, flex the patient's neck, and have the patient swallow.
5. Keep the patient in the upright position while about half of the tube is fed in; then have the patient lie on the right side while an additional 15 to 20 cm are inserted. Less retching will occur if the tube is kept on one side of the pharynx rather than letting it move about. The patient may want to steady it by hand.
6. To check the tube's position, fluoroscope in brief flashes. Radiation exposure will be much less if you tap the foot switch for only brief intervals. You will soon learn to get as much information from a sequence of flashes (still pic-

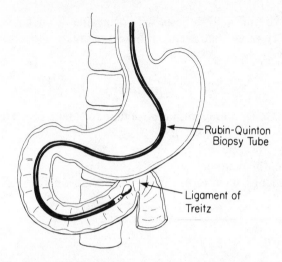

FIG. 1. Configuration of tube for mucosal biopsy at the ligament of Treitz. The tip of the tube is in the correct position when it is a few centimeters left of the spine with the tube in the configuration shown. Occasionally, the tube can double back on itself in the antrum of the stomach and give a somewhat similar appearance even though the tip of the tube remains in the stomach. When there is a question, inject 50–100 ml air through the tube while observing the configuration of the air fluoroscopically. If the location of the tip in the stomach remains a possibility, this can usually be ruled out by fluoroscoping in the lateral position and noting the location of the tip of the tube in the part that is presumably in the C-loop relative to the presumed intragastric portion of the tube. When the position is correct, the latter should be the most anterior as the stomach lies in a plane that is anterior to the duodenum.

tures) as from continuous fluoroscopy (moving picture). Total fluoroscopic time for a biopsy should seldom be more than 90 sec and often less than 30 sec.

7. Luck, art, and science all play a role in getting the tip of the tube to the ligament of Treitz rapidly. A rather firm mercury bolus, approximately 1.3 cm in diameter, in two finger cots on the end of the tube is helpful for small bowel intubation but is usually not needed for biopsy of other parts of the intestinal tract. Three potential problem areas and possible remedies are the following:

a. The tip of the tube lodges on the upper greater curvature shortly after emerging from the gastroesophageal junction. Place the patient in the right lateral decubitus position, withdraw the tube a few centimeters, then advance the tube while an assistant slowly rotates it through 360°.

b. The tip of the tube stops in the area of the pylorus or duodenal bulb:

    i. Force the tip to advance by gentle forward pressure on the oral end of the tube, combined with firm upward pressure on the upper abdomen to prevent a large loop from forming in the stomach. If a coil tends to form in the fundus during this maneuver, rotate the oral end of the tube clockwise or counterclockwise, using the fluoroscope to determine which direction diminishes the tendency to coil.

    ii. With the tip of the tube at the pylorus, inject 20 ml water or air through the tube.

    iii. Give 10 mg metaclopramide intravenously.

    iv. Place the patient in the left lateral decubitus position.

c. The tip of the tube stops in the C-loop at the junction of the second and third portions of the duodenum:

    i. Force the tip of the tube onward until the patient experiences some abdominal discomfort or the tube begins to coil in the stomach. At the same time, deeply massage the abdomen over the tip of the tube to move it medial and superior.

    ii. Place the patient in the left lateral position.

8. Obtain the biopsy when the tip of the tube is in position at the ligament of Treitz (just to the left of the spine):

a. Push the handle in to open the ports.

b. Inject two 10- to 20-ml quantities of air to clear fluid and mucus from the tube.

c. Attach the manometer and syringe.

d. While one person holds the activator handle in (ports open), pull back on the syringe to obtain the desired pressure (see Instruction Manual. We find that the 25-in. Hg pressure recommended for the four-hole instrument causes considerable hemorrhagic artifact and pre-

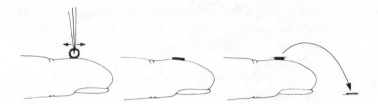

FIG. 2. Orientation of the biopsy specimen prior to fixation. The specimen, which is usually curled as a result of contraction of the cut muscle, must be flattened with the villous side down on the fingertip. This can be done with blunt-tipped pick-up forceps or with the side of a needle. When the specimen is well flattened with the cut side up, a piece of mesh is placed on the cut surface and the specimen is removed from the finger and placed in fixative.

fer to use 12- to 15-in. Hg). If the pressure is not maintained (greater drop than 1 in. Hg in 2 to 3 sec), then there is either an excessive leak in the tube or the mucosa has not been drawn in to occlude the ports.

e. When the pressure has been maintained for 4 sec, the person holding the handles pulls back sharply on the activator handle, cutting off the knuckles of mucosa and closing the ports.

9. Prepare the specimens:

a. Withdraw the tube and place the tip in a Petri dish.

b. Cover the distal ports between the thumb and forefinger and rapidly blow 50 ml air from a syringe through the tube until the specimens in the two upper ports have been blown out into the covered Petri dish.

c. Cover the two upper ports and repeat the process blowing out the specimens from the lower ports.

d. Scoop up the specimens on a dry fingertip with a sweeping motion or with a large blunt pick-up forceps using only surface tension, not pressure, to hold the specimen in the jaws. Usually, the specimen is curled into a ball with the luminal surface outward (Fig. 2). A line can be found where the cut surfaces are in apposition.

e. Gently orient the specimen and flatten it on the fingertip with the cut surface up and the villous surface against the finger. This is done by gently inserting the tip of closed blunt pick-up forceps at the line and allowing the pick-up forceps to open. Alternately, the shaft (not the point) of a needle can be used to open the mucosal ball beginning at the line mentioned.

f. Mount the specimen on monofilament plastic mesh[1] by gently pressing the mesh onto the cut side of the tissue. Remove the fingertip from the luminal surface with a rolling motion. During this maneuver, it may be necessary to hold the biopsy specimen on the mesh with the side of the needle or the tip of the blunt forceps.

g. Immediately put the mounted specimen into paraformaldehyde and record the time on the label.

Postprocedure

1. Instruct patient not to eat or drink until the topical anesthetic has worn off.
2. Instruct patient what to do if gastrointestinal bleeding or severe abdominal pain should occur.

Duodenal Aspiration

The Rubin-Quinton tube with or without the pull wire in place can be used for duodenal aspiration. If the pull wire is in place, be sure to push the handle in to open the ports. If it is not in place, the end of the tube where the activator handle and pull wire usually go must be occluded with a finger or tape to prevent air leak.

Position the tip of the tube in a desired location. To aspirate a sample for giardiasis, the tube should be at least in the third portion of the duodenum. To obtain bile, the tube is placed more proximal in the second portion near the papilla of Vater. Bile secretion is stimulated by instillation of 35 cc 35% magnesium sulfate solution through the tube or intravenous injection of cholecystokinin (0.02 mg/kg). Do not stimulate bile secretion when attempting to aspirate for giardiasis.

---

[1] Plastic mesh may be obtained from National Filter Media Corporation, P.O. Box 156, 969 North Third Street, West Salt Lake City, Utah 84110, Catalog No. 14400399.

Complications

1. Bleeding. One series reported that 4,200 biopsies from the proximal gastrointestinal tract of more than 2,000 patients resulted in only three bleeding episodes, none serious enough to require a transfusion (1).
2. Entrapment of the tube in the duodenum.
3. Bacteremia.
4. Aspiration of fluid or mercury during passage of the tube.
5. Allergic reaction to the local anesthetic.
6. Radiation from fluoroscopy.

Indications for Endoscopically Assisted Duodenal Intubation

When Both Are Needed

When both upper endoscopy and small bowel biopsy are needed, it is usually best to follow the endoscopy with the usual small bowel biopsy procedure. It may be acceptable to obtain several pinch biopsies of the second or third part of the duodenum through the endoscope, using the largest available biopsy forceps (5). In that event, the physician and patient should be prepared for a subsequent formal small bowel biopsy if poor orientation, small size, or crush artifact make the pinch biopsies unsuitable for diagnosis.

When Fluoroscopic Guidance Fails

When duodenal intubation using fluoroscopy fails or is not possible, endoscopic guidance may be indicated. Tie small loops of umbilical tape at 8- to 10-cm intervals beginning near the end of the tube that is to be placed into the duodenum. Pass the tip of this tube into the stomach; then insert the endoscope in the usual manner. Using biopsy forceps through the endoscope, grasp the most distal loop and pass the endoscope and tube into the duodenum. By advancing the biopsy forceps, then successively grasping more proximal loops and advancing the forceps, pass the tube further into the small bowel. If necessary, the same technique is used to keep the tube in place as the endoscope is withdrawn (6).

Other methods for endoscope-assisted duodenal intubation have been published and may be useful in special circumstances. They include passage of small tubes through the biopsy channel of the endoscope (7,8) and insertion of tubes over guide wires passed through the channel of the endoscope (9).

REFERENCES

1. Rubin CE, Dobbins WO (1965): Per oral biopsy of the small intestine. A review of its diagnostic usefulness. *Gastroenterology* 49:676–697.
2. Perea DR, Weinstein WM, Rubin CE (1975): Small intestinal biopsy. *Human Pathol* 6:157–217.
3. Brandborg LL, Rubin GE, Quinton WE (1959): A multipurpose instrument for suction biopsy of the esophagus, stomach, small bowel, and colon. *Gastroenterology* 37:1–16.
4. Linscheer WG, Abele JE (1976): A new directable small bowel biopsy device. *Gastroenterology* 71:575–576.
5. Gillberg R, Ahren C (1977): Coeliac disease diagnosed by means of duodenoscopy and endoscopic duodenal biopsy. *Scand J Gastroenterol* 12:911–916.
6. Chung RSK, Denbesten L (1976): New procedures: Improved technique for placement of intestinal feeding tube with the fibreoptic endoscope. *Gut* 17:264–266.
7. Martin DM, Nasrallah SM (1983): Small intestinal capsule biopsy under endoscopic guidance. *Gastroint Endosc* 29:37–38.
8. Graham MF, Wood R, Halpin TC (1980): Endoscopic small bowel biopsy in children with a modified multipurpose biopsy tube. *Gastroint Endosc* 26:36–37.
9. Mathus-Vliegen EMH, Tytgat GNJ (1983): The role of endoscopy in the correct and rapid positioning of feeding tubes. *Endoscopy* 15:78–84.

11 / Rectal Manometry and Biofeedback Therapy for Fecal Incontinence

Robert S. Sandler

Rectal manometry is a technique used to record pressures from the rectum and the anal sphincters. A major application is in the diagnosis of Hirschsprung's disease, where the internal anal sphincter fails to relax in response to rectal distension (1). Rectal manometry can also be used to evaluate patients with fecal incontinence and for biofeedback conditioning to correct the incontinence (2).

Indications

1. To exclude Hirschsprung's disease in patients with long-standing constipation.
2. Evaluation and biofeedback training for incontinence.
3. Possible diagnosis of scleroderma and dermatomyositis.

Contraindications

None.

Preparation

Generally, no preparation is necessary. If a large amount of hard stool is present or anticipated, administer a Fleet enema.

Equipment

Nonperfused Rectal Manometry Apparatus (Fig. 1)

1. The system consists of a doughnut-shaped balloon that records from the internal sphincter and a pear-shaped bal-

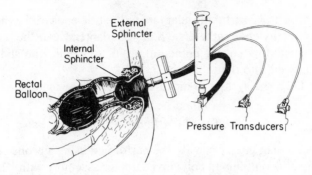

FIG. 1. The apparatus used for rectal manometry is shown in position. Each balloon is linked to a separate pressure transducer. Distension of the rectal balloon with air elicits the rectosphincteric response.

loon that measures pressures from the subcutaneous bundle of the external sphincter.[1]

2. To construct the system, tie the appropriate size balloon to the specially constructed hollow metal cylinder[2] with 4-0 silk sutures. The sutures should be tied over the grooves in the metal cylinder to keep the balloons from sliding. Once the balloons are tied to the cylinder, cut the tip off the balloon.

3. To construct a third balloon for rectal distension, seal the end of a polyethylene tube (file off any sharp edges) and make several holes in the distal closed end with a hot paper clip. The balloon is made by tying a nonlubricated latex condom to the polyethylene tube over the holes. The balloon should have a capacity of 50 cc. It should cover a distance of 3 to 4 cm at the distal end of the tube and have an outside diameter of about 4 cm when distended. The polyethylene catheter from the rectal balloon should pass through the center of the hollow cylinder.

4. Attach polyethylene tubing to the metal tubes that extend from the handle of the metal cylinder.

---

[1] The rectal balloons can be obtained from Affiliated Hospital Products, Perry Division, 1875 Harsh Avenue, S.E. Massillon, Ohio 44646. Catalogue #99501-pediatric size, #99502-intermediate size, #99503-adult size.

[2] The stainless capsules can be obtained from Richard Hiner, 2149 Redthorn Road, Baltimore, Maryland 21220, Catalogue #SS99501-pediatric size, #SS99502-intermediate size, #SS99503-adult size.

5. Attach plastic tubing adapters to the free ends of the three polyethylene catheters. Simple adapters can be constructed by cutting points off a No. 16 needle and sliding the end into the tubing.

6. Check the system to make sure that it is airtight.

Perfused Catheter System

Rectal manometry can also be performed using a probe consisting of a multilumen polyvinyl catheter assembly with 1-mm lateral sensing orifices that are perfused with water by means of a low-compliance pneumohydraulic capillary infusion system. The catheters are similar to those used for esophageal manometry (see Chapter 4) but are modified to include a rectal distending balloon at the distal tip (Arndorfer Medical Specialties, Inc., Greendale, Wisconsin, or Mui Scientific, Mississauga, Ontario, Canada).

Recorder

Any commercially obtained multichannel pen recorder will work. There must be at least three channels, each connected to a pressure transducer.

Additional Equipment

1. Four 50-cc syringes.
2. Exam gloves.
3. A lubricant.
4. Gauze pads, 4 × 4.
5. Towels and gowns.
6. Sterile disposable needle.

Procedure

Nonperfused System

1. Prior to the procedure, make sure that the system is airtight by inflating the sphincter balloons with 10 cc air and the

rectal balloon with 50 cc air for 30 sec. All the air should be recovered if the system is intact.

2. Attach the three polyethylene catheters to the pressure transducers.
3. Lubricate the balloons.
4. The patient should lie on the left side with knees bent. Do a careful rectal exam. Check the anal wink with perianal pinprick using the disposable needle and confirm the patient's ability to voluntarily contract the external sphincter.
5. Insert the apparatus following distension of the anus with a gloved finger.
6. Advance the rectal balloon about 7 to 8 cm.
7. Advance the hollow metal cylinder with its sensing balloons until the external balloon can barely be seen.
8. Inflate the internal balloon with 8 cc air. This will usually pull the apparatus into the rectum and will be felt as a tug on the metal cylinder. If inflation of the internal balloon results in movement of the apparatus out of the anus, deflate the balloon and insert the cylinder a little farther before reinflating.
9. Inflate the external balloon with 8 cc air so that it is partially visible protruding from the anus.
10. Inflate the rectal balloon with 30 cc air two or three times to seat the apparatus and to assess patency of the system.
11. If necessary, adjust the baseline on the recorder so that the tracings are centered.

Internal Sphincter Relaxation

Inflate the rectal balloon with 30 to 50 cc air to evaluate the response of the internal sphincter to rectal distension.

External Sphincter Contraction

Observe contraction of the external sphincter with rectal distension, cough, or perianal pinprick.

Rectal Sensation

Determine rectal sensation by inflating the rectal balloon with 50 cc air and asking the patients if they sense the distension. If the patient recognizes the sensation, decrease the distending volume in 5- to 10-cc increments to determine the *threshold* of rectal sensation. The threshold is the smallest volume of distension sensed.

Perfused System

The technique and equipment used for the perfused system are essentially the same as that used in esophageal manometry, as described in Chapter 4.

1. Calibrate the recording system according to the manufacturer's directions.
2. Inflate the rectal balloon with 50 cc air for 30 sec. All the air should be recovered if the system is intact.
3. Lubricate the balloon.
4. The patient should lie on the left side with knees bent. Do a careful rectal exam. Check the anal wink with perianal pinprick using the disposable needle and confirm the patient's ability to voluntarily contract the external sphincter.
5. Insert the catheter about 10 cm.
6. Slowly withdraw the catheter 0.5 cm at a time using a station pull-through technique similar to that used in esophageal manometry.
7. The pressure will rise as the recording ports enter the anal sphincter. Observe the location, length, and *basal* pressure of the sphincter zone. As the ports are pulled past the sphincter, the pressure will fall to atmospheric.
8. Repeat the pull-through several times to confirm the pressure and location.
9. Insert the catheter into the high-pressure zone and distend the rectal balloon with 30 to 50 cc air. If no reflex relaxation

is seen, check the position of the catheter in the high-pressure zone and repeat.

Maximal Squeeze Pressure

Maximal squeeze pressure can be determined by positioning the catheter in the high-pressure zone and asking the patient to maximally contract the sphincter. The pressure is the absolute pressure recorded during the squeeze. Visual feedback of the recording can sometimes help the patient maximize the response.

Squeeze Increment

This is the difference in pressure between the baseline and maximum pressure recorded.

Rectal Sensation and Sensory Threshold

These are determined by inflating the rectal balloon with air as above.

Postprocedure

1. Wash apparatus in warm, soapy water.
2. Disinfect by soaking in glutaraldehyde solution for 10 min.
3. Apply inert talc to the balloons.
4. Place apparatus in the refrigerator to increase the life of the balloons. With care, balloons may last 6 to 12 months.
5. Recalibrate equipment before the next procedure.

Interpretation

Normal Internal Sphincter Response

In a normal response, the internal sphincter pressure will drop for up to 15 sec. The external sphincter should contract to preserve continence (Fig. 2). Most patients have relaxation down to a distending volume of 15 cc. Several repetitive rectal distensions in rapid succession produce a more pronounced relaxation of the internal sphincter.

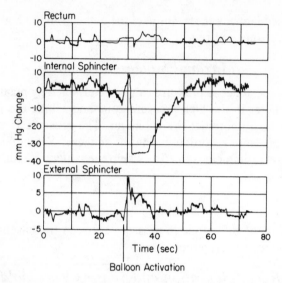

FIG. 2. The normal response to transient rectal distension is shown. The resting pressure of each balloon is assigned a value of zero with relaxation of the internal sphincter and contraction of the external sphincter.

Hirschsprung's Disease

In Hirschsprung's disease, the internal sphincter does not relax after transient rectal distension but, instead, may contract (Fig. 3) (1). The internal sphincter is invariably involved in Hirschsprung's disease. Rectal manometric studies may provide the only means for establishing a diagnosis in short-segment Hirschsprung's disease.

Collagen Disease

In scleroderma, the smooth internal sphincter muscle may fail to relax in response to rectal distension, whereas striated muscle is normal. In contrast, patients with polymyositis have impairment of the external sphincter but a normal internal sphincter (3).

Other Disorders

External sphincter dysfunction has been found in myotonic dystrophy, hypothyroidism, and myasthenia gravis (3). Patients

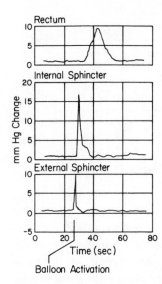

FIG. 3. Manometry response in a patient with Hirschsprung's disease. The internal sphincter contracts instead of relaxing following rectal distension. The external sphincter is normal, but a strong rectal contraction not seen in the normal follows contraction of the sphincters.

with anal fissures may have a characteristic pattern of overshoot contraction of the internal sphincter following a normal relaxation. Rectal manometry is not the first line diagnostic study in any of these diseases.

Muscle Versus Nervous Disorder

The external sphincter response can be initiated by a number of stimuli, such as voluntary effort, postural change, perianal scratch, rectal distension, and increased intra-abdominal pressure (3). If the sphincter responds to any of these, the muscle is intact. If the sphincter fails to respond to all stimuli, there may be either muscle disease or a diffuse neurologic disorder.

Normal Sphincter Pressures

Pressures can be determined by using the perfused system. Because of the broad range of normal pressures, the results must be interpreted in the context of the patient's history and complaints (Table 1).

TABLE 1. Normal Sphincter Pressure Values[a]

Parameter (mm Hg)	Mean	Range
Basal pressure	63 ± 4	24–100
Squeeze pressure	173 ± 14	50–360
Squeeze increment	111 ± 13	18–300

[a] From ref. 4.

Biofeedback Therapy for Fecal Incontinence

Biofeedback refers to techniques in which information about unconscious functions is provided to a patient to gain control over these functions (5). Biofeedback has been applied quite successfully to the problem of fecal incontinence (5,6). Although controlled studies have not been conducted, the technique appears to be promising. There are a number of causes of fecal incontinence including anorectal surgery, spinal surgery, irritable bowel syndrome, rectal prolapse, diabetes, multiple sclerosis, scleroderma, and stroke. Continence has been restored with biofeedback in 70% to 83% of patients, often with one training session (5). The technique is simple, rapid, and without morbidity.

Procedure

1. Perform standard manometry as described above.
2. Show the patient the manometric tracings of the external sphincter.
3. Demonstrate the correct response by drawing it on the tracing.
4. In order to link external sphincter contraction with rectal distension (and relaxation of the internal sphincter), ask the patient to momentarily (2 sec) contract the external sphincter whenever rectal distension is perceived. Distend the rectal balloon with 50 cc air and praise the patient if he appropriately contracts the external sphincter. Progressively decrease the volume of air distension until the sensation threshold is reached.
5. If the sensory threshold is high, progressively decrease the

distending volume in the rectal balloon so that the patient senses smaller volumes and responds appropriately.

6. After conditioning with the recording in view, withhold visual feedback by blocking the patient's view of the tracing.

7. Distensions are performed out of sight of the patient.

8. After the training session, instruct the patient to apply learned techniques consciously for 2 weeks whenever the sensation of rectal distension is felt. Indicate that the reflex will become automatic. For the first few weeks, the patient should practice momentary contractions four times a day.

9. Adding loperamide 2 mg at bedtime may be a useful adjunct to biofeedback. Loperamide increases anal canal pressure and attenuates the rectosphincteric relaxation reflex (7). It also decreases the frequency and looseness of stools. If constipation becomes a problem, the dose can be titrated.

REFERENCES

1. Hirsh EH, Hodges KS, Hersh T, McGarity WC (1980): Anorectal manometry in the diagnosis of Hirschsprung's disease in adults. *Am J Gastroenterol* 74:258–260.

2. Wald A (1981): Biofeedback therapy for fecal incontinence. *Ann Intern Med* 95:146–149.

3. Schuster MM (1973): Diagnostic value of anal sphincter pressure measurements. *Hosp Practice* April:115–117.

4. Schiller LR, Santa Ana CA, Schmulen AC, et al (1982): Pathogenesis of fecal incontinence in diabetes mellitus: evidence for internal-anal-sphincter dysfunction. *N Engl J Med* 307:1666–1671.

5. Marzuk PM (1985): Biofeedback for gastrointestinal disorders: a review of the literature. *Ann Intern Med* 103:240–244.

6. Wald A, Tunguntla AK (1984): Anorectal sensorimotor dysfunction in fecal incontinence and diabetes mellitus: modification with biofeedback therapy. *N Engl J Med* 310:1282–1287.

7. Read M, Read NW, Duthie HL (1980): The effect of loperamide on anal sphincter function. In: *Gastrointestinal Motility,* edited by J Christensen, pp 503–504. Raven Press, New York.

12 / Upper Gastrointestinal Endoscopy

R. Balfour Sartor

Upper gastrointestinal (GI) endoscopy has revolutionized clinical gastroenterology by providing a rapid means of accurate diagnosis and has vast potential for research and therapeutic applications. The purpose of this chapter is to provide an overview of upper GI endoscopy: It is not intended to be a comprehensive source of instruction. Endoscopic technique and interpretation are best taught by an experienced endoscopist, supplemented by a review of recent inclusive texts (1–3) that outline technique in detail.

Indications

The indications for upper GI endoscopy are too numerous to outline completely and must be individualized (4,5). The major indications follow.

Diagnostic

1. To establish the site of upper GI bleeding.
2. To visually define and biopsy abnormalities seen on upper GI series (ulcers, filling defects, and cancers).
3. To evaluate healing of treated gastric ulcers.
4. To evaluate dysphagia, dyspepsia, abdominal pain, and gastric outlet obstruction.

Therapeutic

1. Gastric and esophageal polypectomy.
2. Removal of foreign bodies.
3. Disintegration of bezoars.

4. Coagulation of bleeding points with electrocautery, heat probes, or laser.
5. Sclerotherapy of esophageal varices.
6. Placement of guidewires for esophageal and gastric dilatation.
7. Placement of small intestinal feeding tubes and percutaneous gastrostomy catheters.

Contraindications

Absolute

1. Shock.
2. Acute myocardial infarction.
3. Severe dyspnea with hypoxemia.
4. Coma (unless patient is intubated).
5. Seizures.
6. Acutely perforated ulcer.
7. Atlantoaxial subluxation.

Relative

1. Uncooperative patient.
2. Coagulopathy:
   a. prothrombin time 3 sec over control;
   b. PTT 20 sec over control;
   c. bleeding time >10 min;
   d. platelets <100,000.
3. Zenker's diverticulum.
4. Upper esophageal stricture.
5. Myocardial ischemia.
6. Thoracic aortic aneurysm.

Preparation

1. The patient should have nothing by mouth for 6 to 8 hr prior to the procedure.
2. Review the patient's chart, including X-rays and coagulation studies.
3. See the patient prior to the procedure. Be certain the study

is indicated, that the patient understands the risks and benefits and agrees to the procedure.

4. Write a preprocedure note.
5. Have the nurse or assistant obtain written, informed consent; start the i.v.; and anesthetize the patient's throat with a topical agent.
6. Administer meperidine, up to 50 mg i.v., slowly.
7. If needed, administer diazepam i.v. (1 mg/min) until an appropriate level of sedation is reached. Since the effects of meperidine can be rapidly reversed with naloxone, we prefer this drug to diazepam. Diazepam also has a high incidence of phlebitis, especially when infused into a small vein of the hand. Watch the patient carefully for respiratory depression and give preoperative medication cautiously in elderly and malnourished patients.

Equipment

1. Endoscope of choice. We use the pediatric endoscope routinely and use the large endoscope for anticipated biopsies in patients with gastric ulcers or mass lesions.
2. Light source.
3. Teaching head.
4. Biopsy forceps.
5. Cytology brush.
6. Washing cannula and syringe.
7. Camera.

Procedure

Passing the Endoscope

1. Administer medication so that patient is sedated but alert enough to assist in swallowing.
2. Place the recumbent patient in the left lateral position.
3. Have the assistant hold the scope in a partially flexed (60°) configuration.
4. With the patient's neck partially flexed, pass the endoscope through the hypopharynx, either blindly, using your index finger as a guide, or by direct visualization. For the

latter, insert the tip through the cricopharyngeus, which is seen just posterior to the epiglottis. Use *light* pressure (do not force!) to guide the passage, since forward propulsion is provided by the patient swallowing. With blind passage, be certain to keep the scope in the midline, out of the pyriform sinuses.

5. Once the scope has passed the upper esophageal sphincter (20 cm), advance it under *direct vision* at all times and with only enough air insufflation to permit visualization.

Visualization of Esophagus, Stomach, and Duodenum

1. Advance the scope through the distal esophagus, identifying the gastroesophageal junction by the change from white to coral-colored mucosa ("Z" line) and the lower esophageal sphincter. The level of the diaphragm can be determined by asking the patient to sniff. A hiatal hernia is present if the gastroesophageal junction and gastric folds are significantly above the level of the diaphragm. Barrett's esophagus is identified by an irregular Z line with fingers or islands of gastric epithelium extending into the tan-colored esophageal mucosa.

2. Observe the motility of the stomach, particularly the antrum, for asymmetry and fixation, as subtle invasive lesions are sometimes suspected from damping of gastric contractions.

3. Insert the scope through the pyloric channel into the duodenal bulb, then into the second portion of the duodenum by torquing and turning the tip posteriorly (to the right).

4. The duodenal bulb and pyloric channel are visualized best by slowly withdrawing the scope while rotating the tip by torquing the shaft from side to side. Pay particular attention to the superior and posterior portions of the duodenal bulb.

5. Returning to the stomach, pay special attention to the angulus and the gastroesophageal junction, visualizing both by retroflexion as well as by forward viewing. The endoscope is retroflexed by maximally turning the tip upward so that it is in a J-shape. By rotating the retroflexed scope, the entire gastric cardia can be thoroughly visualized.

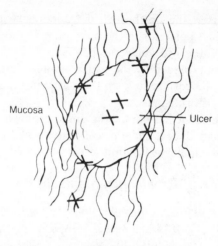

FIG. 1. Sites for biopsying a gastric ulcer. Biopsies (×) should be taken from each of the four quadrants of the margin, the base, and the surrounding gastric mucosa.

6. After thoroughly evaluating the stomach by slowly withdrawing the scope while rotating the tip in a 360° fashion, remove the excess air from the stomach by suction to minimize abdominal distension.

Biopsy

1. It is not necessary to biopsy a routine duodenal bulbar ulcer unless lymphoma is suspected or nodularity or a mass is seen.
2. A gastric ulcer always should be biopsied, unless it is a channel ulcer or prepyloric erosion that is clearly benign. Biopsy the *margin* of the ulcer in all four quadrants, the base several times, and the mucosa next to the ulcer (i.e., at least six to eight biopsies) as demonstrated in Fig. 1. Do not biopsy if the patient has evidence of active or recent bleeding from the ulcer (clot on the base or visible vessel).
3. Do not biopsy the esophageal mucosa if the patient is to have an esophageal dilatation (either Hurst or balloon) within a week of the endoscopy. Use the brush for cytology only.

4. If the biopsy forceps do not pass through the distal channel, straighten the endoscope and try again.

Cytology

Cytologic examination of possible malignant lesions will complement biopsies by increasing their yield of positive results.

Brush Technique

1. Brush suspicious areas several times to obtain adequate cellular material.
2. Stroke the brush over a Dakin slide moistened with normal saline.
3. Place the slide in preservative in a Pap smear bottle.
4. The use of a sheathed brush may produce a better sample by preventing loss of cells in the biopsy channel.

Washing Technique

1. Inject 25- to 30-cc isotonic saline through the biopsy channel onto the lesion.
2. Collect the specimen by aspirating the fluid through the scope into a sputum trap connected to the suction tubing.
3. Send the specimen on ice for immediate processing to prevent lysis of the cells.

Subacute Bacterial Endocarditis Prophylaxis

Prophylaxis is probably indicated for prosthetic valves but not for damaged natural valves (6,7).

1. Aqueous penicillin, 2,000,000 U i.m. or i.v., and gentamicin, 1.5 mg/kg (not exceeding 80 mg) i.m. or i.v. 30 min prior to the procedure and 8 hr postprocedure. Can substitute 2 g ampicillin for penicillin.
2. Penicillin allergies: vancomycin 1 g i.v. and gentamicin 1.5 mg/kg i.m. or i.v. 30 min before procedure and 12 hr later.

Miscellaneous

1. In patients with achalasia, the esophagus should be emptied of retained food prior to endoscopy via a large diameter tube and lavage. This will permit better visualization and prevent aspiration.
2. If esophageal varices are encountered in a patient in whom they are not clinically suspected, make sure they are *carefully* documented by multiple observers and photographs.
3. Rapidly developed photographs can be attached to the procedure note to allow the referring physician to visualize the morphologic findings.

Postprocedure

1. Fill out a procedure sheet and write a summary note in the medical record.
2. Give nothing by mouth until the gag reflex and sensation in the throat return.
3. The patient should not drive for several hours.

Complications

Overall complication rates of the procedure and the medications are in the range of 0.1% to 0.2%, with mortality in the range of 0.014% to 0.065% (8).

1. Drug-induced:
   a. respiratory arrest (0.07%);
   b. phlebitis.
2. Perforation (0.033–0.1%). The most common sites are the pharynx, upper esophagus, and stomach.
3. Bleeding (0.03%). This is from biopsies, dislodging clots from bleeding points, and Mallory-Weiss tears induced by retching during endoscopy.
4. Aspiration (0.08%). The risk can be decreased by giving the patient nothing by mouth, lavaging patients with bleeding or achalasia, and using minimum air insufflation.
5. Retropharyngeal hematomas and crush injuries.
6. Infection:

a. Transient bacteremia (5%). There is only one case report of endocarditis induced by endoscopy.
b. There is no evidence of hepatitis B or acquired immunodeficiency syndrome (AIDS) being transmitted by properly cleaned scopes (9).

7. Complications to the endoscopist:

a. bitten finger;
b. herpetic conjunctivitis;
c. because of the potential transmission of hepatitis and AIDS viruses, we suggest that gloves be worn at all times, particularly in high-risk patients.

REFERENCES

1. Blackstone MO (1984): *Endoscopic Interpretation*. Raven Press, New York.
2. Sugawa C, Schuman BM (1981): *Primer of Gastrointestinal Fiberoptic Endoscopy*. Little, Brown and Company, Boston.
3. Cotton PB, Williams CB (1980): *Practical Gastrointestinal Endoscopy*. Blackwell Scientific Publications, Oxford.
4. Rubin CE, Silverstein FE, McDonald GB (1978): Indications for fiberoptic endoscopy. *Viewpoints Dig. Dis.* 10(5).
5. Grossman MB (1980): Gastrointestinal endoscopy. *CIBA Clin Symp* 32(3).
6. Perucca PJ, Meyer GW (1985): Who should have endocarditis prophylaxis for upper gastrointestinal procedures? *Gastroint Endosc* 31:285–287.
7. Kaye D (1985): Prophylaxis for infective endocarditis: an update. *Annals Int Med* 104:419–423.
8. Shahmir M, Schuman BM (1980): Complications of fiberoptic endoscopy. *Gastroint Endosc* 26:86–91.
9. Villa E, et al (1984): Gastrointestinal endoscopy and HBV infection: no evidence for a causal relationship. *Gastroint Endosc* 30:15–17.

13 / Emergency Upper Gastrointestinal Endoscopy

R. Balfour Sartor

Early esophagogastroduodenoscopy can determine the source of bleeding in upper gastrointestinal (GI) hemorrhage approximately 90% of the time (1,2). It is particularly useful in detecting mucosal lesions that cannot be seen by barium contrast radiography, such as Mallory-Weiss tears, gastritis, and esophagitis (3). However, endoscopy has not been demonstrated to improve the mortality or morbidity associated with routine upper gastrointestinal hemorrhage that ceases spontaneously (85–95% of cases) (4,5), although it may be helpful in continued or recurrent bleeding (1,2). Therefore, *emergency endoscopy should be performed only when it will influence a clinical decision such as medical or surgical therapy.* Otherwise, the procedure can be performed electively with greater safety and improved visualization.

Indications (6)

1. Active upper GI bleeding (recent hematemesis or blood aspirated from the stomach with nasogastric suction).
2. Massive rectal bleeding in which a duodenal ulcer is strongly suspected.

Contraindications

(See Chapter 12, preparation, item 2.) To prevent complications, stabilize the patient hemodynamically prior to the procedure. Be particularly attentive for

1. EKG evidence of ischemia;

2. Hypovolemia;
3. Inability to cooperate; and
4. Severe anemia.

Preparation

1. Decide if the patient is stable enough for endoscopy.
2. Correct severe hypovolemia or anemia with blood transfusions and i.v. fluids.
3. Lavage with large volumes of saline or water using a large tube (Ewald) to remove as many clots as possible. The standard Levine nasogastric tube is inadequate for clot removal. If during the lavage there is no return, do not forcibly aspirate; put in more saline. The gastric mucosa can be traumatized easily by overly aggressive aspiration.
4. Obtain consent for endoscopy and possible therapeutic procedures (esophageal sclerotherapy or coagulation of bleeding site) from the patient or a close relative.
5. Anesthetize the pharynx with a topical agent.
6. Administer premedication (Chapter 12) with greater caution in patients with decreased cardiorespiratory reserve or altered mental status.

Equipment

1. Portable cart for transporting equipment.
2. Endoscope—use an endoscope with a large suction channel to facilitate clot removal and washing.
3. Light source.
4. Teaching head.
5. Camera.
6. Washing cannula and syringe.
7. Sclerotherapy (Chapter 29) and coagulation equipment.

Procedure

1. If possible, arrange for the procedure to be done in the emergency room or intensive care unit, where there is adequate support for the unstable patient.
2. Pass the endoscope in the same manner as for an elective endoscopy (Chapter 12, procedure).

3. Have a nurse or assistant available at all times during the procedure to observe the patient's vital signs and to suction secretions and regurgitated material.

4. After introduction of the scope, inspect the distal esophagus; then go straight to the duodenum, scanning the lesser curvature of the gastric mucosa as you go. The three most important findings are esophageal varices, diffuse gastritis, and duodenal ulcer (treatment is different in varices; surgery should be deferred in diffuse gastritis; surgery is indicated earlier in peptic ulcer disease). Then, if the patient becomes uncooperative, the most important areas will have been seen.

5. Be certain to visualize the gastric cardia by retroflexing the scope to identify Mallory-Weiss tears and gastric varices.

6. Almost always, a large pool of clots will obscure the greater curvature of the fundus. The patient can be rotated on his back or right side to visualize this area better, but extensive pre-endoscopic lavage is well worth the time.

7. Emergency upper endoscopy is not successful in demonstrating the bleeding lesion in 5% to 10% of cases, owing to either clots or active bleeding obscuring the bleeding site or patient noncompliance. In these cases, it is not productive to prolong the procedure and risk aspiration or other complications. It is very helpful to know the approximate location of bleeding and whether diffuse gastritis or varices are present, even if the exact bleeding point is not demonstrated.

8. If there is active bleeding, call a surgeon before endoscopy to see the lesion in order to facilitate early surgery. Treatment of the bleeding lesion with a heat probe, electrocoagulator, laser, or sclerotherapy may be indicated.

9. After a nasogastric tube and gastric lavage, there will almost always be areas of trauma in the fundus. Be cautious of calling erythematous areas gastric erosions when there is no exudate to indicate chronic inflammation.

10. If an ulcer is identified, look for stigmata of recent hemorrhage, indicating a high risk of continued or recurrent

bleeding. These stigmata include a protruding visible vessel, an adherent clot, a black eschar, or actual bleeding (7).

Postprocedure

1. Suction water through the endoscope immediately after the procedure to prevent blockage of the suction channel with clots.
2. Retrieve and clean all equipment.
3. Fill out a procedure sheet and write a summary note in the medical record.

Complications

The risk of major complications in emergency endoscopy is 0.59% (8).

Perforation (0.26%)

Usually involves ulcers.

Aspiration (0.2%)

This is higher than in elective endoscopy because the stomach is full of clots, and the patient's sensorium is frequently diminished.

Hemorrhage (0.13%)

Usually occurs with varices.

REFERENCES

1. Kinard HB III, Powell DW, Sandler RS, Callahan WT, Lapis JL, Levinson SL, Jones JD, Drossman DA, Jackson AL (1981): A current approach to acute upper gastrointestinal bleeding. *J Clin Gastroenterol* 3:231–240.
2. Eastwood GL (1984): Endoscopic diagnosis and management of upper gastrointestinal tract bleeding. *Adv Int Med* 30:449–470.
3. Cello JP, Thoeni RF (1980): Gastrointestinal hemorrhage: Comparative values of double contrast upper gastrointestinal radiology and endoscopy. *JAMA* 233:685–688.

4. Peterson WL, Barnett CC, Smith HJ, Allen MH, Corbett DB (1981): Routine upper endoscopy in upper gastrointestinal bleeding: A randomized controlled trial. *N Engl J Med* 304:925–929.

5. Graham DY (1980): Limited value of early endoscopy in the management of acute upper gastrointestinal bleeding: Prospective controlled trial. *Am J Surg* 140:284–290.

6. Wara P, Stadkilde H (1985): Bleeding pattern before admission as guidelines for emergency endoscopy. *Scand J Gastroenterol* 20:72–78.

7. Storey DW, Bown SE, Swain CP, et al. (1981): Endoscopic prediction of recurrent bleeding in peptic ulcers. *N Engl J Med* 305:915–916.

8. Gilbert DA, Silverstein FE, Tedesco FJ (1981): National ASGE survey on upper gastrointestinal bleeding: Complications of endoscopy. *Dig Dis Sci (Suppl)* 26:55–59S.

14 / Endoscopic Retrograde Cholangiopancreatography

Eugene M. Bozymski

Endoscopic retrograde cholangiopancreatography (ERCP) is a standard procedure used in the diagnosis and treatment of certain diseases of the biliary tree and pancreas. Along with outlining the common bile duct, the intrahepatic ducts, and the gallbladder, we can also visualize the pancreatic ductal system. In addition to a skilled endoscopist, a radiologist with special interest in this area is very helpful in obtaining the maximum information from this procedure.

In cases of obstructive jaundice, the merits of percutaneous transhepatic cholangiography versus ERCP should be debated with respect to the individual patient, keeping in mind the expertise and limitations of the available professional staff. However, there are very few instances in which a gastroenterologist capable of performing ERCP is not readily available.

Indications

1. Evaluation of the patient with suspected obstructive jaundice.
2. Evaluation for suspected disease of the intra- or extrahepatic biliary system.
3. Evaluation of the patient with suspected pancreatic cancer.
4. Evaluation of recurrent pancreatitis of unknown etiology.
5. To determine the anatomy of the pancreas and its ductal system prior to operative, radiologic, or endoscopic intervention for chronic pancreatitis, suspected pancreatic trauma, or pseudocyst or other pancreaticobiliary disorders.

Contraindications

1. Significant bleeding diathesis.
2. Recent acute pancreatitis, unless surgery or endoscopic sphincterotomy is planned for choledocholithiasis.

Preparation

1. Obtain surgical backup.
2. Make certain that there is no barium in the gastrointestinal tract [computed tomography (CT) scan, barium enema] that will obscure the field.
3. All patients having ERCP must be operative candidates.
4. Obtain an informed, written consent.
5. Place an i.v. in the right arm with the port close to the vein for administration of atropine, meperidine, diazepam, or medazolam and glucagon.
6. Have the patient lie on the left side with the left arm behind the back to facilitate the roll to the prone position.
7. Place the patient on preprocedure systemic antibiotics if cholangitis or infection in the pancreatic or biliary tree is suspected. Antibiotic combinations for sepsis frequently used include tobramycin and a newer generation cephalosporin or a third-generation cephalosporin with pseudomonas coverage.

Equipment

1. Duodenoscope.
2. Teaching attachment or television monitoring system.
3. Cannulas filled with renografin (60% for pancreatic duct, 30% or less for biliary tree if small stones suspected).
4. Fluoroscope with spot film cassettes.
5. Lead aprons and thyroid collars.
6. Gloves and lubricant.

Procedure

1. All personnel must wear lead aprons and thyroid collars.
2. Anesthetize the patient's pharynx with a topical anesthetic.

3. Premedicate the patient with 0.4 mg atropine along with meperidine and diazepam or midazolam as needed.
4. Pass the side-viewing duodenoscope; inspect the distal esophagus for varices and rapidly examine the stomach.
5. Identify the pylorus and advance the scope to it.
6. When the pylorus is directly in front of the viewing lens, straighten the tip of the scope so that it can pass through the pylorus in its narrowest diameter, neither flexed nor hyperextended. This is accomplished by viewing the top of the pylorus in the six o'clock position.
7. Enter the pylorus by advancing the scope, noting the distinct "pop" that may be felt as the duodenum is entered.
8. Inspect the duodenal bulb and then rotate the scope 180° clockwise while simultaneously advancing the scope to enter the descending duodenum.
9. Return the scope to its original upright position by counterclockwise rotation. At this point, the descending duodenum will be in view. Frequently, the ampulla of Vater will be visible on the medial aspect of the duodenum. If it is not, examine the duodenum until the ampulla is found. Glucagon may be given in 0.2-cc increments to decrease duodenal motility. If the ampulla is not readily found, it is usually because the scope has descended too far into the second part of the duodenum. Retract the scope while looking for the major papilla as well as any accessory papillas.
10. When the papilla is identified, roll the patient into the prone position to facilitate cannulation and spot filming.
11. Remove any slack in the duodenoscope by pulling it back. This brings the scope along the lesser curvature of the stomach rather than the greater curvature and will usually improve the angle for cannulation, particularly of the bile duct. This "short-sticking" can be accomplished by placing some clockwise torque on the scope and slowly pulling back, angulating the tip of the scope slightly to keep the ampulla at 12 o'clock. As the scope is pulled back to approximately the 60-cm level, the ampulla is brought into position by slight movements of the tip of the scope and body torque.

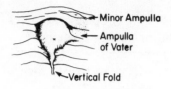

FIG. 1. Major and minor ampulla.

12. Position the ampulla directly in view so that its hood resembles an inverted U with its apex in the 12 o'clock position (Fig. 1). *Do not attempt to cannulate the ampulla until the position is proper.* Any attempt to cannulate without proper orientation usually results in the cannula coming out tangentially. This may also produce trauma to the papilla.

13. Once the papilla is properly positioned, cannulate by advancing the catheter by manipulation of the lever control and rotation of the tip of the scope as well as the actual head of the scope. These manuevers serve to place the tip of the instrument in the proper position. It should be noted that very little movement is necessary during cannulation of the ampulla. Frequent manipulations of the scope, such as advancing and retracting, will lead to patient discomfort and to nausea and vomiting.

14. When the cannula is impacted in the ampulla, advance it for a distance of a few millimeters and inject 1 to 2 cc renografin.

15. Fluoroscope to see which duct is filling.

16. If the pancreatic duct is filling, only 3 to 4 cc dye is needed. Avoid overfilling the pancreatic ductular system. Once lateral branch filling is obtained, stop the injection to *avoid* an acinar pattern. If you are having trouble cannulating the pancreatic duct, remember that it is off to the right of the ampulla and usually toward the bottom and somewhat of a straight shot, compared to the common duct whose entrance is on the upper part of the ampulla to the left side and cephalad. Take films of the pancreatic duct in its entirety.

17. Now, turn your attention to filling the other duct, in this case, the common bile duct. Reinsert the cannula and again inject, and if the common bile duct begins to fill, make

certain that dye is not also going into the pancreatic duct. It may take 15 to 30 cc or more of dye to fill the biliary tree, depending on the presence or absence of the gall-bladder. Make certain that no dye enters the pancreatic duct. Placing the patient in a head-down position at this time may be helpful in filling the proximal intrahepatic ducts. If the cannula is seen to be well into the common duct and there is no filling of the pancreatic duct what-soever, you need not look while injecting dye into the bil-iary tree except at very infrequent levels. *Remember that fluoroscopic time is high exposure time—it is hazardous for patient and staff, and damaging to the fiberoptic bun-dles.* If difficulty is encountered in entering the common duct selectively, you can attempt to place the cannula tip to the upper left portion of the ampulla and try to bow the cannula so that it takes a cephalad position. Take films of the common bile duct as well as all of the intrahepatic radicals. If small gallstones are suspected, use diluted ren-ografin (15–30%) as well as a balloon paddle for compression.

18. With good fluoroscopic imaging, it is frequently possible, after having once entered a duct, to know which duct the cannula is in without repeatedly having to inject dye. This avoids overinjection of the pancreatic ductular system.

19. Once films have been obtained, rapidly remove the scope and take additional films. At this time, further positioning, such as placing the patient supine to view the distal com-mon duct and right hepatic system, may be very useful.

Pancreatic Cytology

If pancreatic cytologies are needed, reposition the cannula in the pancreatic duct and give secretin 1.5 U/kg. Collect pan-creatic secretions over 20 min. Several minutes after secretin is given, pancreatic juice will begin to flow and aspiration can be carried out. If fluid does not come, the cannula may be impacted on the wall, and it should be rotated or moved slightly. Collect the pancreatic secretion in two separate vials. The first will contain a few cubic centimeters of renografin and

FIG. 2. Schematic of the endoscope in "short-sticking" (**A**) and cannulating the minor ampulla (**B**).

should be discarded. The remainder of the pancreatic secretions in the second vial is collected on ice and taken to the cytology laboratory for immediate interpretation.

Helpful Hints

1. If the cannula will not slip into the puncta, change to a tapered one.
2. "Short-sticking" the duodenoscope, i.e., pulling it back into a position along the lesser curve, is preferred since manipulation of the cannula and cannulation of the common bile duct is easier (Fig. 2A).
3. To cannulate the minor ampulla, place the duodenoscope along the greater curvature and use a tapered or metal-tipped cannula (Fig. 2B).
4. Do not try to cannulate from too far a distance; get close to the ampulla and use deliberate, small movements to position the endoscope properly.
5. When a periampullary diverticulum is present, look for the ampulla along the edge.
6. If there is difficulty in finding the ampulla of Vater, it is usually because the operator is beyond it in the descending duodenum.
7. If the axis of the ampulla and puncta is not well aligned for cannulation with the patient in the prone position, change the patient's position to the oblique or lateral.
8. Previous duodenal or bile duct surgery may change the anatomy and pliability of the duodenum and impede cannulation.

Postprocedure

1. Monitor vital signs.
2. When the patient's normal pharyngeal function has returned, clear liquids are permitted and then continued for 24 hr.

3. If there is obstruction to either the pancreatic or biliary tree and the dye does not drain completely from the pancreatic duct or the common bile duct, start the patient on appropriate antibiotics.

Complications

1. Pancreatitis (0.7–7%).
2. Cholangitis (0.65–0.8%).
3. Duodenal perforation (rare).
4. Hemorrhage (rare).
5. Hyperamylasemia without clinical pancreatitis (commonly seen).

BIBLIOGRAPHY

1. Cryan EM, Falkiner FR, Mulvihill TE, Keane CT, Keeling PW (1984): Pseudomonas aeruginosa cross-infection following endoscopic retrograde cholangiopancreatography. *J Hosp Infect* 5:371–376.
2. Dutta SK, Cox M, Williams RB, Eisenstat TE, Standiford HC (1983): Prospective evaluation of the risk of bacteremia and the role of antibiotics in ERCP. *J Clin Gastroenterol* 5:325–329.
3. Geenen JE (1982): New diagnostic and treatment modalities involving endoscopic retrograde cholangiopancreatography and esophagogastroduodenostomy. *Scand J Gastroenterol* 77:93–106.
4. Vennes JA (1977): Technique of ERCP. In: *Atlas of Endoscopic Retrograde Cholangiopancreatography*, edited by E. T. Stewart, J. A. Vennes, and J. E. Geenen, pp. 4–18. Mosby, St. Louis.
5. Bar-Meir S, Geenen JE, Hogan WJ, et al. (1979): Biliary and pancreatic duct pressuress measured by ERCP manometry in patients with suspected papillary stenosis. *Dig Dis Sci* 24:209.
6. Takemoto T, Kasugai T (1979): *Endoscopic Retrograde Cholangiopancreatography*. Igaku-Shoin, Tokyo.
7. Stewart ET, Bennes JA, Geenen JE (1977): *Atlas of Endoscopic Retrograde Cholangiopancreatography*. Mosby, St. Louis.
8. Classen M, Geenen J, Kawai K (1979): *The Papilla Vateri and Its Diseases*. Gerhard Witzstrock Publishing House, New York.
9. Shahml M, Schuman B (1980): Complications of fiberoptic endoscopy. *Gastrointest Endos* 26:86–91.

15 / Colonoscopy

Douglas A. Drossman

Colonoscopy involves examination of the colon and terminal ileum by using a fiberoptic endoscope. Compared to the gastroscope, the instrument is longer, has a larger instrument channel, and is modified to allow greater torque response. The procedure is technically more difficult, requires more patient preparation, and has a slightly greater complication rate than upper gastrointestinal (GI) endoscopy (1)[1].

Indications

As determined by clinical need, patient condition, and cost-effectiveness:

1. Abnormal barium enema examination that requires further evaluation.
2. Occult lower GI bleeding.
3. Gross lower GI bleeding that has stabilized.
4. Pre- or postoperative evaluation of patients with colonic cancer.
5. Screening for colonic cancer in high-risk patients (e.g., ulcerative colitis for more than 10 years, family history of polyposis or cancer).
6. Inflammatory bowel disease, radiation, or ischemic colitis that requires assessment of type or extent of disease (e.g., preparation for surgery).
7. Unexplained chronic diarrhea.
8. Therapeutic. Polypectomy, coagulation of bleeding le-

---

[1] Complications include perforation (0.2%), which occurs most often in inexperienced hands; bleeding (0.1%), usually related to polypectomy; and cardiopulmonary problems (0.04%).

sions, reduction of volvulus or intussusception, decompression of atonically distended colon, dilatation of strictures, removal of foreign bodies.
9. Follow-up evaluation of patients who have had previous polypectomy.

Contraindications

Absolute

1. Peritonitis.
2. Bowel perforation.
3. Toxic or fulminant colitis.
4. Acute diverticulitis.
5. Recent myocardial infarction or pulmonary embolus.

Relative

1. Poor bowel preparation.
2. Inability of patient to physically tolerate or cooperate with the procedure.
3. Recent bowel surgery or history of multiple pelvic operations.
4. Large hernia.
5. Massive colonic bleeding.
6. Unstable cardiopulmonary state (may require monitor and/ or respiratory assistance).

Preparation

Bowel Cleansing

Lavage Solution

Golytely (Braintree Laboratories, Inc., Braintree, Massachusetts 02184) or Colyte (Edlaw Preparations, Inc., 195 B Central Ave., Farmingdale, New York 11735). This has become our standard bowel-cleansing method; it permits excellent visualization, has few side effects, is well tolerated, and does not cause dehydration or fluid overload (2). It is contraindicated in patients with possible intestinal obstruction, bowel perforation, toxic colitis, or megacolon.

1. Low-fiber diet for 48 hr prior to colonoscopy.
2. Clear liquid meal the night before the procedure.
3. 250 cc of prepared solution should be taken orally every 10 to 15 min until at least 1 gallon is consumed. The solution can be made more palatable by adding artificially sweetened flavorings (e.g., Kool-Aid) to the solution. Alternatively, the solution may be given to the inpatient by nasogastric tube.

Standard Bowel Preparation

1. Clear fluids for 48 to 72 hr (3,000 cc/day).
2. 60 cc milk of magnesia two nights before procedure.
3. 10 oz. p.o. magnesium citrate and tapwater enema on night before procedure.
4. Tapwater enema until clear on day of procedure.

Inform the patient of the indications for the procedure, alternative therapy and possible complications. Obtain informed, written consent. Start the i.v.

Bacterial Endocarditis Prophylaxis

Administer bacterial endocarditis prophylaxis if indicated (e.g., prosthetic valve, history of bacterial endocarditis, congenital or rheumatic heart disease, idiopathic hypertrophic subaortic stenosis, surgical systemic-pulmonary shunts). The need for prophylaxis with mitral valve prolapse is not established; in general we do not recommend it. The revised American Heart Association recommendations (3) are as follows:

1. Ampicillin, 2 g i.m. or i.v. and gentamicin 1.5 mg/kg i.m. or i.v., 30 min prior to the procedure and 8 hr postprocedure.
2. Penicillin allergies: vancomycin, 1 g i.v. and gentamicin as above.

3. Oral regimen for low-risk patients: Amoxicillin 3 g orally 1 hr before the procedure and 1.5 g, 6 hr later.

Premedication

Medicate with meperidine up to 25 to 50 mg i.v. slowly until mild sedation or relaxation is achieved. If needed, administer 1 to 3 mg diazepam i.v. (1 mg/min) or midazolam (1 mg). Diazepam may produce phlebitis and excessive respiratory depression in elderly or malnourished patients.

Equipment

1. Colonoscope.
2. Light source.
3. Biopsy forceps, washing cannula, and other accessories as needed.
4. Lubricating jelly (or viscous xylocaine if perianal inflammation present).
5. Gloves, gauze, towels.

Procedure

The following summarizes our use of nonfluoroscopic colonoscopic technique. A more detailed discussion can be found elsewhere (4).

1. Position the patient in the left lateral position. The patient's knees should be drawn up with the buttocks at the edge of the examining table.
2. Perform a rectal examination using two sets of gloves.
3. As the finger is withdrawn, guide the lubricated end of the colonoscope over the finger and advance 3 to 4 cm into the rectum.
4. Remove the outer gloves to avoid greasing the head of the scope.
5. Keep the left-right control partially locked throughout the procedure to maintain torque stability at the tip of the scope.
6. Control tip deflection and scope passage with the right hand grasping the insertion tube near the anus. Remove the hand

only to reposition the left-right controls at the head of the scope.

7. Let the colonoscope hang toward the floor with the right thigh bracing the insertion tube (at about 20 cm from the anus) against the table. This prevents the scope from slipping out of the rectum when the right hand is removed and "shortens" the scope length to permit easier passage control.

8. Position the left hand on the head of the scope so that the thumb can freely move the up-down controls.

9. Visualize the rectum. Usually, a "red-out" is first seen; withdraw the instrument 1 to 2 cm and insufflate air until the mucosa and lumen are seen.

10. Advance the scope under direct visualization, directing the tip as much as possible with torque maneuvers by the right hand.

11. *Use of torque.* This is a technique for advancing the scope around bends. It causes stiffening of the tube and with the controls locked, also turns the tip of the scope. In the region of the sigmoid a counterclockwise spiral is usually made. After that, lesser degrees of clockwise torque are needed to get around the flexures. When the lumen angulates behind a fold, torque the scope so the tip turns into the lumen and advance it.

12. Relubricate the anal area whenever resistance occurs.

13. *Technique in difficult situations.* When uncertain of what to do or where the scope tip is located, make frequent use of withdrawing movements. When no lumen is seen, withdraw and "jiggle." A jiggle is a series of rapid in-and-out movements with torque directed toward the lumen. If a crescent is seen indicating lumen behind it, turn the scope into the crescent and jiggle while gradually withdrawing. This sheaths the bowel on the scope, straightens it, and tends to move the lumen into view (Fig. 1). *Do not* advance (push) if a loop is being made (determined by paradoxical movement or less than a 1:1 response of the tip-to-tube passage from the rectum) if you cannot see lumen or if resistance to passage occurs. In these situations, the following maneuvers may be tried:

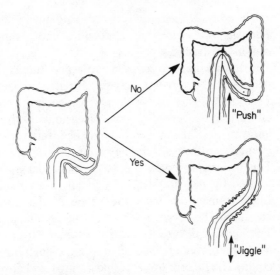

FIG. 1. Techniques for advancing the endoscope in difficult situations. Pushing the endoscope through areas of angulation tends to form loops. A series of gentle but rapid in-and-out motions sheaths the colon on the endoscope and tends to straighten the bowel, thus permitting advancement.

    a. Jiggle the tube.
    b. Straighten the tube by withdrawing.
    c. Change the position of the patient. For example, place the patient supine when the hepatic flexure is reached.
    d. Suck out air. This tends to shorten the bowel and advance the tip. This is most successful on the right side of the colon.
    e. Apply abdominal pressure. Downward pressure on the sigmoid colon loop in the left lower quadrant tends to straighten it; upward midabdominal pressure straightens the transverse colon.
    f. In some cases, pushing through the loop may afford progress, although it produces greater patient discomfort.

14. Remain aware of intracolonic landmarks:
    a. The *rectum* has prominent bluish vessels. The semilunar valves of Houston are usually seen on withdrawal of the instrument.

b. The *rectosigmoid angulus* occurs at about 15 to 17 cm.

c. The *sigmoid colon* has concentric and symmetrical ring-like valvulae.

d. The *descending colon* is narrow and tubular in appearance; the valvulae may be absent.

e. The dome of the *splenic flexure* is seen at the proximal end of the descending colon. Occasionally, the bluish impression of the spleen is seen. The transverse colon is entered after a sharp angulation.

f. The *transverse colon* has large, thin triangular folds formed by the lateral muscle bands, the taeniae coli. Light transmitted from the scope in the transverse colon may be seen anywhere on the abdomen.

g. The *hepatic flexure* is seen just after the liver imparts a bluish colored appearance to the proximal transverse colon. The flexure traverses posteriorly and downward for about 10 cm and will transilluminate the patient's right flank.

h. The *ascending colon* has asymmetric folds, and the lumen is quite large. It will illuminate the right upper and lower abdominal quadrants.

i. The *cecum* can be identified when
    i. the light is transmitted through the skin just above the right inguinal ligament;
    ii. the terminal ileum, appendiceal lumen, and sling fold of the caput cecum ("Mercedes Benz" sign) are identified;
    iii. a lumen cannot be visualized (least reliable).

j. Sometimes, pushing with one finger on the abdomen and noting the area of greatest indentation through the scope is helpful.

15. *Cannulation of the ileum.* The ileocecal valve is not well visualized, as it is directed downward into the cecum (Fig. 2A). It is usually found medially behind a flat, rolled fold located just before entering the cecum and 3 cm above the terminal portion of the cecum. Cannulation is best accomplished by advancing the scope beyond the fold, turning into the fold, and slowly withdrawing the scope while gently torquing the shaft back and forth (Fig. 2B). Often

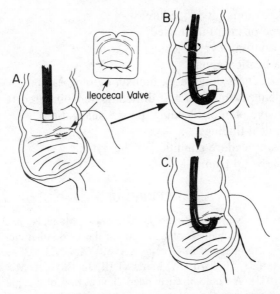

FIG. 2. Cannulation of the ileocecal valve. The valve orifice is directed downward and away from the endoscope. Cannulation can be accomplished by (**A**) advancing the endoscope beyond the fold, (**B**) turning into the fold and slowly withdrawing the scope while gently torquing the shaft back and forth. The tip will "pop" through the valve and advance into the ileum (**C**).

the tip will "pop" through the valve, and it can then be advanced into the ileum (Fig. 2C).

16. Perform a thorough examination of the colon when withdrawing from the cecum. *This is the most important part of the procedure.* Check behind folds and examine carefully the lesser curvatures. The natural tendency on withdrawing is for the scope to straighten, thereby visualizing mainly the greater curvatures.

17. When the rectum is reached, the endoscope can be retroflexed to examine for hemorrhoids, papillitis, fissures, or other anorectal disorders.

Postprocedure

Be certain that the patient's condition is stable. Write a brief postprocedure note in the medical record containing the following:

1. Indications for procedure.
2. Type of instrument used.
3. The visual level reached.
4. Medication given.
5. Procedures done (e.g., biopsy, cytology).
6. Adequacy of prep and difficulties encountered (e.g., excessive pain or bleeding, poor visualization).
7. Clinical findings.
8. Postprocedure condition of the patient.
9. Follow-up plan.

REFERENCES

1. Silvis SE, Nebel O, Rogers G, Sugawa C, Mandelstam P (1976): Endoscopic complications. Results of the 1974 American Society for Gastrointestinal Endoscopy survey. *JAMA* 235:928–930.
2. Ernstoff JJ, Howard DA, Marshall JB, Jumshyd A, McCullough AJ (1983): A randomized blinded clinical trial of a rapid colonic lavage solution (Golytely) compared with standard preparation for colonoscopy and barium enema. *Gastroenterology* 84:1512–1516.
3. Shulman ST, Amren DP, Bisno AL, et al (1984): Prevention of bacterial endocarditis: a statement for health professionals by the Committee on Rheumatic Fever and Infective Endocarditis of the Council on Cardiovascular Disease in the Young. *Circulation* 70:1123A–1127A.
4. Waye JD (1981): Colonoscopy intubation techniques without fluoroscopy. In: *Colonoscopy. Techniques, Clinical Practice and Colour Atlas*, edited by RH Hunt and JD Waye, pp. 147–178. Chapman and Hall, London.
5. Shinya H, Wolff WI (1976): Colonoscopy. *Surg. Ann.* 8:257–295.

16 / Flexible Sigmoidoscopy

Robert S. Sandler

The flexible sigmoidoscope is a fiberoptic instrument that is designed to examine the rectum and sigmoid colon. The instrument was developed in order to correct several of the deficiencies of the rigid sigmoidoscope. It was thought that the flexibility of the instrument would provide patients with a more comfortable exam and that the longer length would compensate for the more proximal location of benign and malignant tumors of the large bowel. These goals have generally been met. Although there remains some controversy about its precise role, many believe that the flexible sigmoidoscope will replace the rigid scope as the primary diagnostic instrument for detecting colorectal disease (1).

Indications

Routine screening for colon cancer in those over age 50.

Minor Bright-Red Rectal Bleeding

Although the flexible sigmoidoscope will not localize bleeding below 20 cm any better than the rigid scope, it may reveal other pathology in the rectosigmoid above the reach of the rigid instrument. Bleeding from an anal fissure or internal hemorrhoid is easily missed, so anoscopy should also be employed to evaluate patients with bright-red rectal bleeding. Unexplained lower gastrointestinal bleeding or iron-deficiency anemia requires full colonoscopy.

Sigmoid Volvulus

A volvulus can be reduced with a rigid or flexible instrument but will often recur if not corrected surgically.

Postoperative Bowel Resection

To examine the anastomosis for stricture, bleeding, or recurrent tumor.

Inflammatory Bowel Disease

To monitor disease activity when full colonoscopy is not needed; to evaluate patients with acute colitis.

Adjunct to X-Ray

To evaluate lesions seen on X-ray within reach of the instrument; to examine the rectosigmoid where lesions can be missed on X-ray.

Physical Incapacity

Since the exam is performed in the lateral position, it is useful in the elderly and those with debilitating illnesses, cardiac decompensation, and broken limbs.

Pseudomembranous Colitis

Although pseudomembranous colitis will sometimes spare the distal bowel, examination with the flexible sigmoidoscope will reveal 90% of cases (2).

Postradiation

To differentiate radiation colitis from cancer; for screening in order to reliably examine the entire radiated segment.

Contraindications

The contraindications to flexible sigmoidoscopy are to some extent relative. They must be balanced against the potential information that the study will provide.

1. Acute peritonitis.
2. Fulminant colitis/toxic megacolon.
3. Uncooperative patient.
4. Acute, severe diverticulitis.

Preparation

1. A single Fleet enema given 5 to 20 min prior to the exam will provide adequate preparation in 80% to 90% of cases. Outpatients may take the enema at home 1 to 2 hr before the procedure.
2. Obtain informed, written consent.
3. Although the exam can usually be performed without sedation, some patients will require intravenous sedation.

Equipment

Flexible Sigmoidoscope

There are a number of instruments available (2). They vary in length from 35 to 72.5 cm, and have either two-way or four-way tip deflection. Air and water feeding may be manual or automatic. The shorter instrument was designed for the generalist (3). Because of its shorter length, it was felt to be safer, better tolerated by patients, and easier to master. Some have found that the pathology found is comparable to that with the longer instrument (4). Although the 65-cm instrument may be more difficult to use, in certain patients its longer length may be an advantage.

Other Equipment

1. Light source.
2. Suction apparatus.
3. Biopsy forceps and cytology brush.
4. Gloves.
5. Lubricant.
6. Gown for patient and operator.
7. Permit form, result sheet.
8. Water for irrigation.
9. Luer-tip syringe, 50 cc.

Procedure

The technique of flexible sigmoidoscopy is similar to that of colonoscopy (see Chapter 15). Although descriptions of the

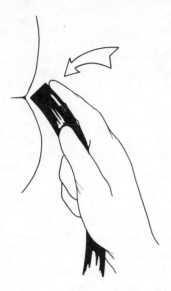

FIG. 1. Correct 90° wedged insertion.

technique can be found in the literature (2,5), there is no sub-stitute for training under the supervision of a skilled endoscopist.

1. Place the patient in the left lateral decubitus position.
2. Do a careful rectal exam. If stool is encountered, admin-ister another enema.
3. Examine the anal canal and distal rectum with an anoscope before sigmoidoscopy in patients with symptoms localized to the anal area.
4. Lubricate the distal 10 to 15 cm of the instrument. Do not get lubricant on the lens. Make sure that the air and suction are operating adequately.
5. Insert the instrument into the anus as the gloved finger is withdrawn or gently insert the tube obliquely by pressing the curved surface of the tip against the sphincter, rather than straight on (Fig. 1).
6. The tube can be advanced by the examiner or by the as-sistant. The tip should be deflected to keep the lumen in view as the instrument is advanced. Use as little air as possible, since air distension stretches the colon, making

the exam more difficult and more uncomfortable for the patient.

7. When the lumen is not seen, pull the scope back a few centimeters. The pattern of folds as the bowel collapses behind the withdrawing endoscope will indicate the proper direction of passage. If the colon is in spasm, as indicated by puckered folds, apply gentle bursts of air to distend the lumen.

8. For the beginner, simply advance the tube until it will go no further with gentle pressure. Technical maneuvers to advance the scope further should be reserved for those with more experience. The goal is to provide a safe, thorough, and comfortable exam and not to insert the instrument to its full length.

9. If the tube will not advance around the rectosigmoid junction (at about 15 cm), gentle pressure will sometimes open the angle and permit the scope to pass. This maneuver is safe, even if the lumen is not clearly seen ahead, as long as the mucosa slides by. If the patient is uncomfortable or if the scope does not advance, stop the procedure or try rotating the shaft of the scope (torque).

10. Torque may be applied with short scopes by rotating the control head of the scope and with longer scopes by twisting the shaft itself near the anus. Gentle clockwise torque is often effective to help advance the scope, find the lumen, and straighten angulated bowel. By pulling the scope back while applying torque, loops in the bowel can be straightened.

11. Moving the tube in and out a few centimeters at a time (jiggling, dithering) may also sleeve the bowel onto the scope. This advanced maneuver, which is often effectively combined with torque, is described in greater detail in Chapter 15.

12. The bowel is best examined on slow withdrawal of the instrument. The tip should be methodically deflected behind each valve and fold. Air insufflation, torque, and tip deflection can be used on withdrawal. Endoscopic pinch biopsies should be taken of any lesions seen. Biopsies should always be taken under direct vision.

13. To prevent explosions, coagulation biopsies (hot biopsies) or snare electrocautery should not be attempted unless the patient has had a full colonoscopic prep.

Postprocedure

1. Review the findings with the patient.
2. The patient may resume normal activities immediately.
3. If biopsies were taken, caution the patient that small quantities of blood may be seen in the stool.

REFERENCES

1. Hogan WJ (1983): Flexible sigmoidoscopy—when to use which instrument. *Gastrointest Endosc* 29:126–128.
2. Katon RM, Keefe EB, Melnyk CS (1985): *Flexible Sigmoidoscopy*. Grune & Stratton, Orlando.
3. Winawer SJ, Cummins R, Baldwin MP, Ptak A (1982): A new flexible sigmoidoscope for the generalist. *Gastrointest Endosc* 28:233–236.
4. Zucker GM, Madura MJ, Chmiel JS, Olinger EJ (1984): The advantages of the 30-cm flexible sigmoidoscope over the 60-cm flexible sigmoidoscope. *Gastrointest Endosc* 30:59–64.
5. Hocutt JE, Jaffe R, Owens GM, Walters DE (1982): Flexible fiberoptic sigmoidoscopy. *American Family Physician* 26:133–141.

17 / Anoscopy and Rigid Sigmoidoscopy

Don W. Powell

The increased use of flexible sigmoidoscopy to examine the rectum and distal colon has not alleviated the need for the physician to become proficient in the use of the anoscope and rigid sigmoidoscope. Most gastroenterologists believe that the anal canal is still most optimally evaluated with the anoscope. The anoscope and rigid sigmoidoscope are still the instruments of choice if the physician is only interested in the distal 15 cm of the alimentary canal (e.g., when considering hemorrhoids or proctitis as a cause of rectal bleeding, following the disease course of patients with known proctitis, or when evaluating the anorectum for conditions such as fistula-in-ano or perirectal abscess). In addition, rigid sigmoidoscopy can be performed anywhere there is an electrical outlet, with largely disposable equipment that does not require expertise for cleaning or maintenance, and without the need for specially trained ancillary personnel. To ensure the most complete examination of the colorectum and the anus, anoscopy could be performed in conjunction with either flexible sigmoidoscopy or colonoscopy.

Indications (1–5)

1. Symptoms referable to the colon, rectum, or anus: bleeding, discharge, protrusions or swellings, pain—either abdominal or anorectal, diarrhea, constipation or a change in bowel habits, severe itching.
2. Unexplained fever.
3. Patient evaluation prior to anorectal surgery.
4. To observe the progression or regression of colorectal disease.

5. To obtain tissue for histological study or stool and/or exudate for bacteriologic or parasitologic study.
6. To evaluate the rectum in any patient in whom a barium enema is to be performed.
7. As a routine part of the physical examination, although the age at which this is to begin and the frequency of such an examination, as well as the cost-effectiveness, remain controversial.

Contraindications

There are no absolute contraindications to proctosigmoidoscopy.

1. Since patients with heart disease have an increase in ectopic beats with sigmoidoscopy, cardiac monitoring and/or awareness of possible arrhythmias in these patients is advised (6).
2. Since bacteremia occurs in 10% of patients undergoing sigmoidoscopy (7), antibiotic prophylaxis (including coverage for the enterococcus) is advised in patients with valvular or congenital heart disease who are at risk (see Chapter 15, Colonoscopy).

Preparation

1. Most patients can and should be examined with no prior preparation.
2. If stool precludes an adequate examination, a Bisacodyl Suppository or Fleet enema can be given and the examination carried out 1 hr later.
3. In rare circumstances, a tap water or saline solution enema given at bedtime the night before and then repeated the next morning 3 to 4 hr prior to examination will be necessary for optimal visualization.
4. Premedication (sedation) is rarely necessary, although intravenous meperidine and/or diazepam can be useful in unusual circumstances.

Equipment

Minimal Equipment

1. An anoscope and sigmoidoscope. An adult sigmoidoscope is adequate for all but the infant.
2. Cotton swab sticks.
3. An examination table or bed.
4. A sheet to cover the patient.
5. Gloves, lubricant, and 4 × 4 gauze pads.

Useful Equipment

1. Sigmoidoscopy table.
2. Suction.
3. Air insufflator.
4. Sigmoidoscopy spoon.
5. Biopsy tools: either alligator type (see procedure section, Rectal Biopsy with Alligator Forceps), colonoscopic biopsy forceps taped to a stick or suction-type biopsy capsule.
6. Epinephrine solution and silver nitrate sticks.

Procedure

Be gentle and reassuring throughout the procedure. Inform the patient what is to be done. Advise the patient that a few deep breaths during the examination will often relax muscles and sphincters.

Position

Position the patient for the examination (2,3).

Left Lateral (Sims') Position

This is best for bedridden or feeble patients or to assess anal pathology such as hemorrhoids. Be sure to get buttocks to the edge of the bed or table by placing the patient diagonally across the bed (Fig. 1a).

Knee-Chest Position

This is adequate for most examinations. It requires more patient stamina and cooperation (Fig. 1b).

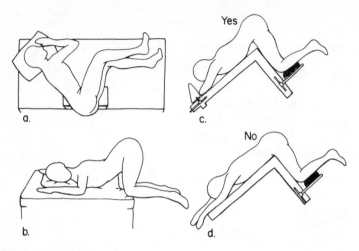

FIG. 1. Three major positions for anoscopy and sigmoidoscopy. **a:** Left lateral (Sims') position. **b:** Knee-chest position. **c:** Prone, inverted (jack-knife) position. **d:** An improper jackknife position is shown; the knee rest is too low, and no elbow rest is provided.

Prone Inverted (Jackknife) Position with Sigmoidoscopy Table

This is the most comfortable position for the patient and the examiner (Fig. 1c). Place the patient's knee rest high enough so that the "broken" table does not compress the abdomen. This allows the pelvic organs to "fall away" when the sigmoidoscope is advanced. Elbow rests are preferred so that the patient does not slide off the end of the table (Fig. 1d).

Digital Examination

Inspect the perianal area and perform a digital examination.

1. If two gloves are worn on the examining hand, some decrease in sensitivity of touch is experienced; but time is saved, since the soiled glove can be stripped off, and one can proceed with anoscopy or sigmoidoscopy.
2. Spread the buttocks apart and inspect the perineum for cutaneous or anal pathology.

3. Palpate the perianal and perineal tissues for abscesses or fistulae.
4. Perform the digital exam with a well-lubricated finger. The digital exam relaxes the anal sphincters and facilitates insertion of the scope. Try to palpate any abnormalities you wish to visualize at anoscopy. Sweep the finger circumferentially around anal canal; a blind spot to sigmoidoscopy is directly posterior and proximal to the anal ring. Examine anteriorly for cul-de-sac lesions; do not mistake the cervix for tumor. Stool from the examining finger can be checked for occult blood.

Anoscopic Examination

Perform anoscopic examination (4–6). The anoscope is most useful to view fissures, fistula openings, internal hemorrhoids, papillitis and cryptitis, and neoplasm.

1. Insert either a clean plastic anoscope or a metal anoscope with a slotted end. It should be warm and well lubricated.
2. Stabilize the obturator with the thumb and insert by aiming toward the umbilicus.
3. After inserting 3 to 4 cm, move the tip posteriorly.
4. If anal spasm is encountered, ask the patient to bear down or breathe through the mouth.
5. If the slotted metal anoscope is used, do not rotate the inserted scope. Remove it, replace the obturator, and then reinsert the scope each time you wish to view a different quadrant.
6. Visual examination of hemorrhoids with the anoscope is facilitated by having the patient strain (Valsalva) as you remove the anoscope. This is particularly important in the knee-chest position, where internal hemorrhoids may collapse.

Sigmoidoscopy Examination

Perform sigmoidoscopic examination (4–6). We prefer the clear plastic disposable sigmoidoscope to the reusable metal one.

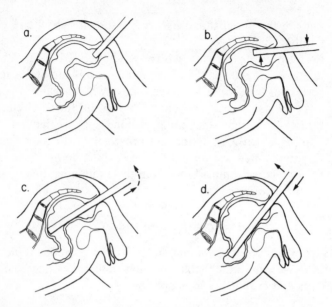

FIG. 2. Sequence of steps of the sigmoidoscopy. **a:** Sigmoidoscope, with obturator, is inserted, aimed toward the umbilicus. **b:** With the obturator removed, the tip of the scope is rotated posteriorly and advanced. **c:** If the lumen is lost, the sigmoidoscopy is retracted until the lumen is found and **(d)** then advanced.

1. Introduce the sigmoidoscope blindly only for the first 3 to 5 cm while stabilizing the obturator with the thumb. Aim toward the umbilicus (Fig. 2a). Remove the obturator and, from this point on, advance the sigmoidoscope under direct vision.

2. Swing the tip of the sigmoidoscope posteriorly to follow the curve of the sacrum (Fig. 2b). Advance the scope as far as possible.

3. If the lumen is lost, the end of the sigmoidoscope is probably occluded by a valve or the rectal wall or is at the rectosigmoid junction (Fig. 2c). Do not push forward! Pull back 2 to 3 cm, rotate the scope until the lumen reappears, and then advance (Fig. 2d). Often, the tip of the advancing scope can "iron out" a fold or curve and aid in passage. Some examiners insufflate air if the lumen cannot be visualized; however, this may increase the postprocedure dis-

comfort. The rectosigmoid junction is encountered at 12 to 15 cm, and many sigmoidoscopies will end here. Often, this point can be negotiated by straightening the bend with the end of the scope or by insufflating air.

4. Withdraw the scope slowly, rotating the tip circumferentially to observe the entire rectal wall. Check the stool from this point for occult blood. Also test the mucosa for friability. Twirl a swab on the mucosa; then remove it and observe for capillary bleeding. Look behind the rectal valves of Houston.

Rectal Biopsy with Alligator Forceps

1. Unless a specific lesion is to be biopsied, the *posterior* rectal mucosa should be biopsied below the peritoneal reflection (within 7–10 cm of the anal verge) to lessen the chance of free peritoneal perforation.
2. Biopsies from the free edge of a valve are technically the easiest, but the large biopsy obtained increases the chance of bleeding or perforation. Biopsy from the base of the valve is probably safer.
3. Bleeding can usually be stopped by applying pressure with a dry cotton or with epinephrine-soaked swabs (1 ml of 1:1,000 epinephrine diluted 1 to 10 with saline fluid).
4. After the bleeding has halted, the biopsy site may be cauterized with silver nitrate sticks.

Postprocedure

The patient may resume normal activity. Inform the patient that some "gas pains" may be experienced, but to notify you if persistent pain or bleeding occurs.

REFERENCES

1. Schrock TR (1978): Examination of the anorectum, sigmoidoscopy, and colonoscopy. In: *Gastrointestinal Disease: Pathophysiology, Diagnosis, Management*, edited by MH Sleisenger and JS Fordtran, pp 1548–1559, 2nd ed. WB Saunders Company, Philadelphia.

2. Goligher JC, Duthie HL, Nixon HH (1980): *Surgery of the Anus, Rectum, and Colon*. Baillière Tindall, London.
3. Otto P, Ewe K (1979): *Atlas of Rectoscopy and Colonoscopy*. Springer-Verlag, Berlin.
4. Turell R (1960): Proctosigmoidoscopy. *The New Physician*, 9:23–28.
5. Castro AF (1960): Diagnosis and management of common rectal and anal disorders. *Am Fam Physician* 34:78–92.
6. Fletcher GF, Earnest DL, Shuford WF, Wenger NK (1968): Electrocardiographic changes during routine sigmoidoscopy. *Arch Intern Med* 122:483–486.
7. LeFrock JL, Ellis CA, Turchik JB, Weinstein L (1973): Transient bacteremia associated with sigmoidoscopy. *N Engl J Med* 289:467–470.

18 / Secretin Injection Test for Diagnosis of Gastrinoma

Robert S. Sandler

The diagnosis of gastrinoma (Zollinger-Ellison syndrome) can generally be made by demonstrating elevation in serum gastrin and increased acid secretion in a patient with ulcer disease. If the fasting gastrin is greater than 1,000 pg/ml and gastric acid secretion is elevated, the patient almost certainly has a gastrinoma (1). However, there may be substantial overlap in serum gastrin and acid secretion between patients with gastrinoma and those with common peptic ulcer. Approximately 40% of patients with proven gastrinoma have fasting gastrins from 100 to 500 pg/ml, which is similar to the range seen in ulcer patients without gastrinomas (2). In order to increase the accuracy of diagnosis, a number of provocative tests have been devised (3). The secretin injection test is the most reliable and easiest to do (1).

Indications

Patients in whom the diagnosis of gastrinoma is suspected but not established or excluded.

Contraindications

None known.

Preparation

1. The patient should be fasting for 12 hr.
2. Although cimetidine has not been convincingly shown to

affect serum gastrin (4), it is reasonable to stop H_2-blocking agents (cimetidine, ranitidine) 10 to 12 hr prior to the secretin test.

Equipment

1. Large-bore (No. 18 or larger) angiocath.
2. Seven small blood-collection tubes with labels to indicate the time the samples are drawn.
3. Basin of ice.
4. Sterile three-way stopcock.
5. Intravenous (i.v.) tubing and bag of i.v. solution (D_5W).
6. Secretin-Kabi (Pharmacia Laboratories) 2.0 U/kg. Do *not* use Boots secretin, which has been associated with false-positive increases in serum gastrin (5).
7. Eight 3-cc syringes.
8. Electric timer.
9. An assistant.

Procedure

1. Start a large-bore i.v. in an antecubital or other large vein.
2. Connect the angiocath to the tubing via the three-way stopcock.
3. Clear the angiocath of all i.v. solution by drawing a small quantity of blood and discarding it prior to collecting each sample.
4. Obtain baseline samples 10 min and 1 min before injection of secretin (1). Place samples on ice immediately.
5. Give 2.0 U/kg secretin by bolus injection over 30 sec.
6. Collect 3-cc samples at 2, 5, 10, 20, and 30 min (1).

Postprocedure

Remove the i.v.

Interpretation

More than 90% of patients with a gastrinoma will have an increase in gastrin, usually at 2 or 5 min (1). Although there have been several criteria that have been suggested (2), an absolute increase of 200 pg/ml is generally regarded as diagnostic (1). There may be occasional false negatives using this criterion, but false positives have not occurred. In normal individuals, those with duodenal ulcer disease, or those with antral G-cell hyperplasia, i.v. secretin either decreases or has no effect on serum gastrin levels. Some patients with duodenal ulcer and hypersecretion with no evidence of gastrinoma may have an increase in gastrin level after secretin (6), but the increase is less than 200 pg/ml.

REFERENCES

1. Jensen RT (1983): Differential diagnosis and provocative test. In: Jensen RT, moderator. Zollinger-Ellison syndrome: current concepts and management. *Ann Intern Med* 98:59–75.
2. Ippoliti AF (1977): Zollinger-Ellison syndrome: provocative diagnostic tests. *Ann Intern Med* 87:787–788.
3. Wolfe MW, Jain DK, Edgerton JR (1985): Zollinger-Ellison syndrome associated with persistently normal fasting serum gastrin concentrations. *Ann Intern Med* 103:215–217.
4. McGuigan JE (1981): A consideration of the adverse effects of cimetidine. *Gastroenterology* 80:181–192.
5. Brady CE, Johnson RC, Williams JR, et al (1979): False positive serum gastrin stimulation due to impure secretin. *Gastroenterology* 76:1106.
6. Malegelada J-R, Glanzman SL, Go VLW (1982): Laboratory diagnosis of gastrinoma. II. A prospective study of gastrin challenge tests. *Mayo Clin Proc* 57:219–226.

19 / Bentiromide Test for Diagnosis of Exocrine Pancreatic Insufficiency

Ray L. James, Jr.

The bentiromide test is an orally administered noninvasive screening test for exocrine pancreatic insufficiency. Bentiromide (Chymex, Adria Laboratories) is cleaved by the pancreatic enzyme chymotrypsin liberating p-aminobenzoic acid (PABA), which is absorbed, conjugated by the liver, and excreted by the kidneys into the urine. The amount of PABA excreted can be determined by measuring the total urinary arylamine concentration. Since patients with exocrine pancreatic insufficiency have low levels of chymotrypsin available to cleave the bentiromide, less PABA is absorbed, and urine levels are decreased.

Indications

1. To diagnose exocrine pancreatic insufficiency.
2. To monitor the adequacy of supplemental pancreatic enzyme therapy.

Contraindications

1. Patients with a known allergy to PABA.
2. Patients taking methotrexate, since PABA displaces methotrexate from binding sites.
3. Safe use during pregnancy, in nursing mothers, or in children under 6 years old has not been established.

Preparation

1. Give nothing by mouth after midnight.
2. Discontinue 3 days before the test:

   a. Drugs that are metabolized to arylamines—

Acetaminophen	Chloramphenicol
Phenacetin	Procainamide
Benzocaine	Sulfonamides
Lidocaine	Thiazides
Procaine	

   b. Multivitamin or sunscreen preparations containing PABA.

   c. Prunes or cranberries from the diet.

3. Discontinue any pancreatic enzyme supplements for 5 days before the test.
4. Do not repeat the test for 7 days.

Procedure

1. Have patient void immediately before drug administration.
2. For adults, administer orally 500 mg bentiromide (1). For children, administer orally 14 mg/kg body weight (2).
3. Have the patient drink 250 ml water initially and at least another 250 ml within the first 2 hr of administration (3).
4. An additional 500 ml water or more may be given in hours two through six to stimulate urine flow (1).
5. Collect all urine for 6 hr, being sure that the patient voids at the 6-hr mark to complete the collection. Record the urine volume.
6. Refrigerate a 10-ml aliquot for analysis.
7. Submit the sample to a lab capable of performing the Smith modification of the Bratton-Marshall test for arylamines.[1]

---

[1] National Medical Services, 2300 Stratford Ave., Willow Grove, Pennsylvania 19090. Smith, Kline and French (formerly Bioscience), 1777 Montreal Circle, Tucker, Georgia 30084.

Postprocedure

Resume usual diet and medication.

Complications

None known, although there is the potential for allergic reactions to bentiromide or PABA.

Interpretation

1. The recovery of the PABA in the urine is determined by the following formula:

$$\% \text{ PABA recovered} = \frac{(\text{mg PABA/ml})(V)(2.95)}{\text{mg bentiromide administered}}$$

   where mg PABA/ml is calculated by lab and corrected for dilution; V is urine volume from 6-hr collection; and 2.95 is the conversion factor. (Most labs will calculate the percent PABA recovered if the value for V and the bentiromide dose is supplied to them.)
2. A normal PABA excretion is greater than 57% (2). The smaller the value, the greater the likelihood of pancreatic insufficiency. Some patients with mild or even moderate pancreatic exocrine insufficiency may fall within the 50% to 75% range. All results less than 50% should be considered abnormal. A bar graph is available for further interpretation (Fig. 1).
3. False-positive tests (i.e., excretion less than 50%) may occur in patients with Billroth II gastrojejunostomy, small intestine disease, liver disease, kidney disease, or diabetes mellitus. The specificity of the test may be improved by calculating a PABA excretion index after oral administration of either PABA (on a separate test day) or ^{14}C-PABA (same day as bentiromide) (4). This variation of the bentiromide test is not routinely used.
4. The test does not differentiate between chronic pancreatitis, pancreatic cancer, or other potential causes of exocrine pancreatic insufficiency (5).

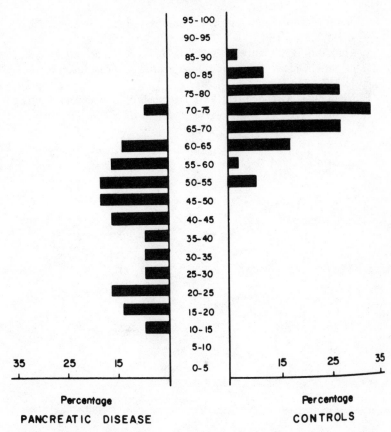

FIG. 1. Relative frequency distribution of urinary arylamines for patients with pancreatic disease and control subjects. Note overlap in 50% to 75% range (2).

REFERENCES

1. Toskes PP (1983): Bentiromide as a test of exocrine pancreatic function in adult patients with pancreatic exocrine insufficiency: determination of appropriate dose and urinary collection interval. *Gastroenterology* 85:565–569.
2. Nousia-Arvanitakis S, Arvanitakis C, Desai N, Greenberger NJ (1978): Diagnosis of exocrine pancreatic insufficiency in cystic fibrosis by the synthetic peptide N-benzoyl-L-tyrosl-*p*-aminobenzoic acid. *J Pediatrics* 92:734–737.
3. Chymex (bentiromide): An oral screening test for exocrine pan-

creatic insufficiency. Adria Laboratories, Inc, Columbus, Ohio 43215.
4. Lankisch PG, Lembcke B (1984): Indirect pancreatic function tests: chemical and radioisotope methods. *Clin Gastroenterol* 13:717–737.
5. Niederau C, Grendell JH (1985): Diagnosis of chronic pancreatitis. *Gastroenterology* 88:1973–1995.

20 / Abdominal Paracentesis

Henry R. Lesesne

Aspiration and examination of peritoneal fluid has been an important diagnostic procedure for many years in the differential diagnosis of ascites and acute abdomen and in the evaluation of blunt trauma to the abdomen.

Indications

1. Evaluation of ascites.
2. Detection of perforated viscus in a patient with an acute abdomen or following blunt trauma to the abdomen.

Contraindications

1. Disorders of blood coagulation:
   a. prothrombin time >5 sec of control;
   b. platelet count <50,000 mm^3.
2. Intestinal obstruction.
3. Infection of the abdominal wall.
4. Relative contraindications:
   a. poor patient cooperation;
   b. history of multiple abdominal surgeries;
   c. portal hypertension with abdominal collateral circulation.

Preparation of Patient

1. Obtain hematocrit, prothrombin time, and platelet count at least 48 hr prior to procedure.

2. Explain the risks, benefits, and details of the procedure to the patient.
3. Obtain written consent.

Equipment

1. Sterile gloves.
2. Betadine and alcohol; sterile gauze.
3. Draping towels.
4. Local anesthetic (lidocaine, 1%) and needles.
5. Syringes: 10 cc × 2; 50 cc × 2.
6. Paracentesis needles:
   a. 16, 18, 20 gauge;
   b. spinal needle (18, 20 gauge) for obese patients;
   c. intravenous catheter with polyethylene tubing (18 gauge).
7. Sterile specimen tubes.
8. Glass slides × 2–3.
9. Specific gravity hygrometer.
10. For removal of >250 cc fluid (e.g., for therapeutic paracentesis):
    a. Bard-Parker blade (No. 11).
    b. Paracentesis trocar and stylet (14 gauge).
    c. Polyethylene tubing (PE-190/512), 12 to 18 cm in length, 16 gauge.
    d. Three-directional stopcock.
    e. Rubber tubing.
    f. Sterile container, 1 liter.
    g. Absorbable suture with needle.

Procedure

Diagnostic Paracentesis

1. Have patient empty bladder.
2. Position the patient in the bed with the head elevated 45° to 90°. This allows fluid to accumulate in lower abdomen. (If there is a small volume of ascitic fluid, the patient can be asked to assume the knee–hand position on the side of the bed with the physician working from below.)

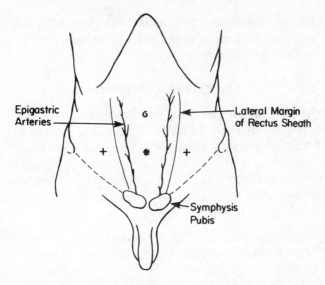

FIG. 1. Various sites for paracentesis: (*) preferred; (+) secondary.

3. Identify the point of aspiration; in the midline midway between the umbilicus and pubic bone (Fig. 1). If scars from previous surgeries are present, choose the right or left lower quadrant lateral to the rectus muscles.
4. Put on sterile gloves.
5. Sterilize the site with Betadine and then alcohol.
6. Place sterile draping towels.
7. Inject lidocaine down to and including the peritoneum.
8. Attach an 18-gauge needle (spinal needle for obese patients) to a 10-cc syringe and insert this into the peritoneal cavity and inject 5 cc air.
9. Gently aspirate 10 cc fluid, and then attach 50-cc syringe and aspirate further quantities of fluid as needed for predetermined analysis (see below).
10. If no fluid returns on aspiration, insert intravenous catheter into peritoneal cavity and gently thread polyethylene tubing into the cavity. Remove the needle and gently aspirate fluid using a 10-cc syringe. You may shift the patient around to find small amounts of fluid. The knee–hand position may help in this situation.

11. Remove the needle (or catheter) and place a Band-Aid or pressure dressing over the site. The patient may resume normal activities.

Therapeutic Paracentesis

When the patient's ascites is causing respiratory difficulties, pain, or hemodynamic difficulties, removal of 750 to 1,000 cc fluid may be indicated. Recently, large-volume paracentesis (5 liters) has been reintroduced as a safe therapeutic option in the patient with tense ascites (2). If needed, central venous pressure monitoring should be available to guard against significant depletion of intravascular volume.

1. Prepare the patient and give local anesthetic as described.
2. Make a 2-mm incision at the site with a No. 11 Bard-Parker blade.
3. Insert the 14-gauge trocar and stylet into the peritoneal cavity; remove the stylet and flush with 5 cc air.
4. Thread the polyethylene tube through the trocar and attach to a three-directional stopcock.
5. Attach a 50-cc syringe and to the lateral arm of the stopcock attach rubber tubing, which is then inserted into the sterile, 1-liter bottle.
6. Aspirate 50 cc fluid at a time and then inject into the large bottle.
7. Remove the polyethylene tubing.
8. Using absorbable sutures, close the incision and apply Band-Aid or pressure dressing.
9. Monitor vital signs and/or central venous pressure for 6 hr following procedure.

Analysis of Fluid

The analysis of the aspirated fluid will be determined by the individual patient and his/her diagnosis. Routine tests employed include the following (3,4):

1. Specific gravity of ascites (hygrometer at bedside). If specific gravity is over 1.020, one should suspect exudative ascites.

2. Total protein and albumin (4).
3. Red and white blood cell count.
4. Gram and AFB stains.
5. Amylase.
6. Culture (bacterial, AFB, fungal).
7. Cytology (at least 50 cc).
8. Others chemistries as indicated: CEA, LDH, triglyceride, cholesterol, etc.

Complications

The incidence of serious complications from paracentesis is unknown. One study of 242 diagnostic paracentesis in patients with liver disease recorded seven major complications, including serious hemorrhage and perforation of the bowel (5).

REFERENCES

1. Streckler JH, Ervin PD, Rice CO (1958): Diagnostic paracentesis. *Arch Surg* 77:859–863.
2. Kao HW, Rakow NE, Savage E, Reynolds TB (1985): The effect of large-volume paracentesis on plasma volume—a cause of hypovolemia? *Hepatology* 5:403–407.
3. Boyer TD, Reynolds TB (1978): Diagnostic value of ascites fluid, LDH, protein, and white blood cells. *Arch Intern Med* 138:1103–1105.
4. Rector WG Jr, Reynolds TB (1984): Superiority of serum-ascites albumin difference over ascites total protein concentration in separation of "transudative" and "exudative" ascites. *Am J Med* 77:83–85.
5. Mallory A, Schaefer JW (1978): Complications of diagnostic paracentesis in patients with liver disease. *JAMA* 239:628–630.

21 / Percutaneous Peritoneal Biopsy

Henry R. Lesesne

Needle biopsy of the peritoneum is a useful adjunct to the evaluation of a patient with unexplained ascites. Percutaneous biopsy using the Cope needle is simple and inexpensive. At times, direct peritoneal biopsy during peritoneoscopy is indicated. (Most of the information in Chapter 20, Abdominal Paracentesis, applies here.) The following specifically relates to the percutaneous biopsy of the peritoneum using the Cope needle.

Indications

Peritoneal biopsy should be considered to rule out tuberculosis, fungal infection, and metastatic carcinoma in a patient with exudative ascites, particularly when bacterial cultures and cytology are negative.

Contraindications

1. Prothrombin time >3 sec.
2. Platelets, <50,000 mm^3.
3. Portal hypertension with evidence of collateral circulation.

Equipment

1. Equipment used in therapeutic paracentesis (see Chapter 20).
2. Cope needle (trocar, biopsy shaft, and snare).
3. Formalin solution for fixation of tissue.

Preparation

See Chapter 20.

Procedure

1. Prepare the patient and give local anesthetic as described.
2. Do not attempt this procedure if ascitic fluid is not easily aspirated with the anesthetic needle.
3. Make a 2-mm skin incision at the biopsy site. Levine (1) prefers biopsying in the left lower quadrant (see Fig. 1, Chapter 20).
4. Introduce the biopsy shaft and trocar into the peritoneal cavity.
5. Have the assistant apply pressure to the contralateral side of the abdomen to create a large cushion of fluid in the operating area.
6. If fluid is needed for further examination, remove the trocar and aspirate.
7. Introduce the snare (needle) attached to a syringe through the biopsy shaft and withdraw the snare until it engages the peritoneum.
8. Complete the biopsy by rotating the biopsy shaft forward over the snare.
9. Remove the snare.
10. Fix the tissue in formalin or place in sterile container with sterile saline for culture.
11. Repeat the procedure three or four times with the tip of the snare in different directions to obtain several samples.
12. Close the incision with absorbable sutures and apply a pressure dressing.
13. Send the biopsy specimens in the labeled formalin jar to the laboratory.

Postprocedure

1. Monitor vital signs for 6 hr (q.1 hr).
2. Keep the patient at bedrest for 6 hr.

REFERENCE

1. Levine H (1967): Needle biopsy of peritoneum in exudative ascites. *Arch Intern Med* 120:542–545.

22 / Percutaneous Liver Biopsy

Henry R. Lesesne

Percutaneous liver biopsy has been a widely accepted procedure for the study of liver disease for the past 40 years. Because it is a potentially hazardous, invasive procedure, it should be undertaken only after initial noninvasive studies of the liver disease have been nonproductive or suggest a need for examination of liver tissue. Outpatient liver biopsy can be considered if appropriate facilities are available (1,2). Difficult cases (small liver, unsuccessful blind biopsy) can be aided by computed tomography (CT) or ultrasonic localization (3). When tense ascites or severe coagulation is present, transvenous needle biopsy may be considered (4).

Indications

1. To diagnose suspected primary liver disease or unexplained hepatomegaly.
2. To assess the course of certain liver diseases (e.g., chronic active hepatitis) and response to therapy.
3. To confirm the presence of malignant disease.
4. To assist in the diagnosis and staging of lymphomas.
5. To assist in the diagnoses of metabolic disease (e.g., glycogen storage disease), multisystem disease (e.g., sarcoidosis, tuberculosis, or hemochromatosis), or pyrexia of unknown origin. (Biopsies may be cultured and stained for specific organisms.)
6. To assess the effect of hepatotoxic drugs (e.g., methotrexate in treatment of psoriasis).

Contraindications

1. Uncooperative patient.
2. Abnormal clotting parameters:

   a. prothrombin time >3 sec of control;
   b. PTT >20 sec of control;
   c. TCT >4 to 5 sec of control;
   d. platelet count <100,000/mm^3;
   e. prolonged bleeding time (>10 min).

3. Severe anemia, hematocrit <30.
4. Local infection:

   a. infected pleural effusion;
   b. peritonitis (ascites should be cultured prior to biopsy).

5. Massive, tense ascites.
6. High-grade extrahepatic obstructive jaundice.
7. Severe uremia (BUN >50).

Preparation

To be done prior to the procedure.

1. Prebiopsy checklist:

   a. Check patient's general condition and coperation.
   b. Obtain Hct, BUN, PT, PTT, TCT within 48 hr of biopsy.
   c. Obtain bleeding time.
   d. Review chest film (look for pleural effusion or, rarely, bowel under right diaphragm).
   e. Review liver scan if obtained.
   f. Send clot to blood bank: "Type and screen—liver biopsy tomorrow."

2. Explain the procedure including benefits, risks, and alternatives; have consent form signed and witnessed.
3. Write prebiopsy note to include:

   a. Statement of indication for liver biopsy.
   b. Statement of any contraindications to biopsy. Explain if any relative contraindications exist and note precautions that will be taken.

4. Write orders for procedure:

  a. Nothing by mouth after midnight.
  b. The following to be at bedside in the morning:

    i. Liver biopsy tray.
    ii. Two pairs of gloves size ____.
    iii. Betadine, alcohol, and 1% lidocaine.
    iv. Six 5-cc vials sterile saline.
    v. Sterile bottles for cytology and culture specimens.
    vi. Band-Aid.
    vii. 4% Paraformalin solution for fixation of specimen.

  c. To empty the gallbladder, have the patient drink a carton of milk at 7 A.M.

Equipment

The liver biopsy tray should include the following (see Preparation, item 4,b):

1. Klatskin or Menghini liver biopsy needle (16 gauge).
2. Petri dish.
3. No. 11 blade and holder.
4. Gauze.
5. Forceps.
6. Syringes (10 cc × 2).
7. Punch to make hole in skin to allow needle to pass.
8. Spinal needle (22 gauge) to determine depth of diaphragm from skin.
9. Sterile towels.

Procedure (5, 6)

Position Patient

Position patient near edge of bed with right arm under the head and left arm by left side.

Identify Site for Liver Biopsy (Fig. 1)

1. Slightly posterior to midaxillary line.
2. Two finger-breadths below the upper border of hepatic

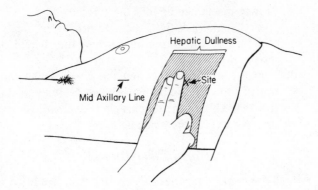

FIG. 1. Percutaneous liver biopsy.

dullness *or* midway between the upper and lower borders of hepatic dullness.
3. Above the bottom rib of the intercostal space.

Teach patient to hold his/her breath at end-expiration while using your finger to simulate the needle stick.

Sterilize Biopsy Area

1. Wash hands and put on sterile gloves.
2. Cleanse the area thoroughly with Betadine or other cleansing solution. Begin at the biopsy site and wash with an expanding circular motion.
3. Repeat in the same manner using alcohol.
4. Drape the patient with sterile towels.

Prepare Site for Biopsy

1. Infiltrate needle tract through skin, subcutaneous tissue, and diaphragm with 1% lidocaine. The tract should be *horizontal* to the bed and about 5° off the perpendicular in the direction of the xiphoid.
2. With the punch (or No. 11 blade), make a small incision in the skin (this will allow easy passage of the liver biopsy needle).
3. With the spinal needle, find the depth of the diaphragm:

a. Slowly insert needle into the tract.
b. Every 5 mm, ask the patient to breathe.
c. You are in the *diaphragm* when the needle head moves downward.
d. You are in the *liver* when the needle head moves upward toward the patient's head. Note the distance from the skin to the diaphragm (~1–2 cm) for placement of liver biopsy needle.

Perform Liver Biopsy

1. Attach the liver biopsy needle to a 10-cc syringe filled with saline fluid.
2. With the measurement taken by the spinal needle as a guide, insert the liver biopsy needle to the diaphragm. Be certain you are past the rib so that it will not be hit during the actual biopsy.
3. Flush 1 cc saline fluid through needle to clear it of skin or fat.
4. Ask patient to take in a breath, blow it *all out*, and hold in end-expiration.
5. Grasp the needle with your left hand 2.5 cm from skin. This is your *guard*.
6. With your right hand, produce negative pressure by withdrawing syringe plunger 1 to 2 cc (for cirrhosis, use 3-cc suction).
7. In one motion, push syringe and needle in 2.5 cm (to finger guard) and come out quickly. Suction should be maintained at all times. This "1-sec technique" will allow the liver specimen to be aspirated into the saline fluid-filled syringe.
8. If bleeding occurs, apply direct pressure to puncture site with sterile gauze.
9. At least 2.5 cm of liver tissue is needed for examination. A second or third biopsy should be performed for more tissue, and especially to minimize sampling error (e.g., chronic hepatitis, metastatic liver disease).

Fix Liver Specimen

1. Express 1 cc of fluid through the needle to remove any tissue remaining in needle.

2. Remove the syringe plunger and allow the tissue specimen and saline fluid in the syringe to flow into the Petri dish.
3. Decant the excess saline fluid from the Petri dish without disturbing the liver specimen.
4. Pour the paraformalin solution into the Petri dish to fix the specimen.

Have the patient slowly turn onto the right side. The patient should be able to move his or her arms and legs while keeping constant body pressure on the biopsy site for 2 hr. The next 22 hr will be spent at bedrest, or, if the patient has been stable for 12 hr, bathroom privileges can be allowed with nurse assistance.

Cytology

1. Inject fluid aspirated from the Petri dish into the sterile specimen bottle.
2. Send fluid for cytology.

Culture[1]

1. Leave a small amount of saline fluid in sterile specimen bottle along with a small piece of liver (0.5–1.0 cm).
2. Cover sterile bottle.
3. Send sterile bottle to microbiology lab for routine, AFB, and fungal cultures as needed.
4. If viral cultures desired, place small piece of liver in appropriate medium at the bedside.

Histopathology

1. Return the liver specimen and formalin to the specimen bottle.
2. Send to histopathology lab, noting the time the specimen was fixed.

---

[1] Culture specimens should be obtained *prior to* fixation of the specimen.

Postprocedure
Procedure Note

Write procedure note. Include what was done, location of the biopsy site, how many "passes" were made, where the specimens were sent, and give a description of the liver specimen.

Post-Liver-Biopsy Orders

Write post-liver-biopsy orders. Suggested format:

1. Strict bed rest for 24 hr; first 2 hr on right side. Patient may sit up after 12 hr.
2. Blood pressure, pulse: every 15 min × 2 hr; every 30 min × 2 hr; every 1 hr × 8 hr; *then* every 4 hr until breakfast in the morning.
3. Notify physician on call if blood pressure <90/60, pulse >110, severe pain.
4. Diet: clear liquids for 6 hr, then full liquids for 18 hr. Resume regular diet in 24 hr.
5. Obtain venous hematocrit in 6 hr.

Post-Liver-Biopsy Note

Write a post-liver-biopsy note (6 and 24 hr postbiopsy):
1. Statement of condition of patient and any complications noted.
2. If possible, attach photograph of liver biopsy and report preliminary findings.

REFERENCES

1. Perrault J, McGill DB, Ott BJ, Taylor WF (1978): Liver biopsy: complications in 1000 inpatients and outpatients. *Gastroenterology* 74:103–106.
2. Westaby D, Macdougall BRD, Williams R (1980): Liver biopsy as a day-case procedure—selection and complications in 200 consecutive patients. *Br Med J* 281:1331–1332.
3. Bjork JT, Foley WD, Varma RR (1981): Percutaneous liver biopsy in difficult cases simplified by CT or ultrasound localization. *Dig Dis Sci* 26:146–148.

4. Lebrec D, Goldfarb G, Degott C, Rueff B, Benhamou JP (1982): Transvenous liver biopsy. *Gastroenterology* 83:338–340.
5. Edmondson HA, Schiff L, Schiff ER (1982): Needle biopsy of the liver. In: *Diseases of the Liver*, edited by L Schiff and ER Schiff, pp 303–331. JB Lippincott Co, Philadelphia.
6. Sherlock S, Dick R, Van Leeuwen DJ (1984): Liver biopsy today— the Royal Free Hospital experience. *J Hepatol* 1:75–85.

23 / Peritoneoscopy (Laparoscopy)

Henry R. Lesesne

Until recently, peritoneoscopy has been of limited use in internal medicine. It is now considered one of the most reliable techniques available for closing the gap between clinical evaluation and surgical exploration (1).

Indications

1. Guided liver biopsy under direct visualization.
2. Guided biopsies of the peritoneum to aid in the evaluation of ascites.
3. Assessing operability among patients with proven carcinoma.
4. Staging of lymphomas.
5. Evaluation of intra-abdominal masses.
6. Evaluation of suspected pelvic pathology.
7. Evaluation of patients with acute and chronic abdominal pain.

Contraindications

1. Poor patient cooperation (general anesthesia may be considered).
2. Disorders of blood coagulation:
   a. prothrombin time, >3 sec of control;
   b. PTT, >20 sec of control;
   c. TCT, >4 to 5 sec of control;
   d. platelet count, <100,000/mm^3;
   e. bleeding time, >10 min.
3. Hematocrit, <30.

4. Peritonitis.
5. Intestinal obstruction.
6. Infection of abdominal wall.
7. Relative contraindications:
   a. severe cardiac or pulmonary disease;
   b. large abdominal hernias;
   c. history of multiple abdominal surgeries (adhesions will decrease visualization and increase risk of perforation);
   d. tense ascites.

Preparation of Patient

1. X-ray and laboratory studies:
   a. obtain Hct, BUN, prothrombin time, PTT, TCT, and bleeding time, at least 48 hr prior to procedure;
   b. obtain and review chest X-ray, KUB, ECG.
   c. type and cross for 2 U of whole blood or packed red cells;
   d. culture of ascitic fluid;
   e. review liver scan and/or CT scan (if available).
2. Explain the risks, benefits, and details of the procedure to the patient.
3. Have patient sign consent form.
4. Write a preperitoneoscopy note to include
   a. statement of indication for procedure;
   b. statement that there are no contraindications, or explanation of the relative contraindications, detailing the precautions to be taken;
   c. orders—
      i. nothing by mouth following midnight;
      ii. begin intravenous fluids (D_5W) at 8 A.M;
      iii. Fleet enema at 8 A.M;
      iv. on call to procedure, have patient empty bladder;
      v. abdominal shave, if there is excessive hair growth around the umbilicus.

Equipment[1]

1. Fiberoptic projector with light-transmitting cable.
2. N_2O automatic insufflator with tubing.
3. Verres cannula for pneumoperitoneum.
4. Operating peritoneoscope and accessory instruments:
   a. cannula with trumpet valve and trocar;
   b. operating scope;
   c. biopsy forceps;
   d. liver biopsy needle for scope.
5. Second puncture instrument with biopsy forceps.
6. Standard liver biopsy tray to be used for guided liver biopsy using the percutaneous approach.
7. Accessories for procedure:
   a. draping towels ($\times 6$);
   b. Betadine and alcohol;
   c. syringe, 10 cc $\times$ 3 to 4; 50 cc $\times$ 1;
   d. Needles for local anesthetic;
   e. Bard-Parker blade (No. 11);
   f. absorbable suture; Steristrips;
   g. local anesthetic (Marcaine or Xylocaine, 1%);
   h. hemostats ($\times 6$), forceps $\times 2$;
   i. scissors;
   j. gauze sponges.

Procedure

Peritoneoscopy may be performed in a well-equipped endoscopy suite that contains resuscitation equipment. Physician trainees should learn this procedure in the operating room with an experienced peritoneoscopist in attendance. An assistant is needed to obtain biopsies. A surgeon should be on call or available for any complications.

1. With patient supine, infuse meperidine, 25 to 50 mg slowly (naloxone should be available for respiratory depression);

[1] Recommended peritoneoscopy equipment and accessories are made by American Cytoscope Makers, Inc.; Eder Instrument Company; Storz Instrument Company; and Richard Wolf Instrument Company.

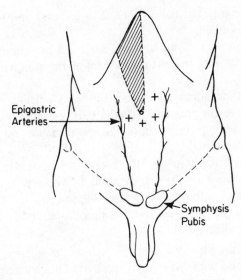

FIG. 1. Various sites for insertion of peritoneoscope; (*shaded area*) falciform ligament.

then infuse diazepam (1 mg/min) until slurred speech or horizontal nystagmus occurs.

2. Put on a mask and surgical gown and hand scrub for 5 min. Put on sterile gloves.

3. Sterilize the abdomen with diluted Betadine from nipples to pubis with center of sterilization around umbilicus. (This large area allows for a second puncture during procedure.)

4. Inject local anesthetic down to and including the peritoneum. The site for insertion of instrument is shown in Fig. 1. Avoid areas of previous surgery, enlarged organs, the falciform ligament, and the epigastric vessels. If cirrhosis is present, collateral veins may form around the umbilicus—insertion should be done with caution and possibly in the left upper quadrant in such circumstances.

5. Make a 5-mm horizontal incision with the Bard-Parker blade and insert the Verres (pneumoperitoneum) needle into the peritoneum, with the patient tensing his or her abdomen with a Valsalva maneuver.

6. Infuse nitrous oxide (N_2O, 2 to 3 liters) and remove the Verres needle.

7. Extend the incision to about 1.0 to 1.5 cm (enough to allow cannula with trocar to pass through the skin without causing N_2O leakage).

8. Insert the cannula with trocar during a Valsalva maneuver.

9. Remove the trocar. Place the peritoneoscope in the cannula and pass it into the peritoneum under direct visualization.

10. Systematically inspect the abdominal contents, noting the appearance of the peritoneum, pelvic organs, intestine, mesentery, liver, spleen, and diaphragm.

11. Biopsy procedures (to be done only after full inspection of the abdomen):

    a. *Liver*. The liver can be biopsied through the operating scope with either the special liver biopsy needle or forceps (for accessible, focal lesions). Biopsy can also be performed using the percutaneous liver biopsy needle inserted over the liver with guidance by the peritoneoscopist. Likewise, the second puncture instrument can be inserted over the liver and focal lesions biopsied with forceps. Local anesthetic should be sprayed over the liver (or peritoneum) using tubing inserted through the peritoneoscope prior to biopsy.

    b. *Peritoneum*. Guided peritoneal biopsy can be done with the scope forceps or with the second puncture instrument and forceps.

    c. *Other structures*. Mass lesions involving other organs (mesentery, spleen, stomach wall, pancreas) can be biopsied with forceps, being careful not to biopsy highly vascular lesions or pulsating masses.

12. Aspirate ascitic fluid for culture and cytologies as needed.

13. To complete the procedure:

    a. Remove the scope. Allow N_2O to escape by asking the patient to do several Valsalva maneuvers.

    b. Remove the cannula.

    c. Close the incision with two to four subcutaneous absorbable sutures. Cover with Band-Aid. Steristrips or suture may be used to close second puncture instrument incision.

14. Processing of biopsy material: The biopsy material should be handled as explained in the Liver Biopsy Procedure (see page 152).

Postperitoneoscopy Procedure

1. The patient should be returned to the room with orders written as in Liver Biopsy Postprocedure (see page 154). The dictated operative note should include:

   a. preoperative diagnosis;
   b. postoperative diagnosis and findings;
   c. operation;
   d. attending physician, assistants;
   e. anesthesia used;
   f. specimens (pathology, cytology);
   g. cultures;
   h. estimated blood loss.

   A summary of these findings should be recorded in the chart.

2. Continue intravenous fluids for 24 hr at a "keep-open" rate.

3. The physician should evaluate the patient at 6 and 24 hr postprocedure, assessing for signs of active bleeding or peritonitis and recording any notable findings. (*Note.* A small amount of N_2O may remain and cause minimal abdominal pain. Mild analgesia may be used.)

4. The patient may be discharged after 24 hr.

Equipment Sterilization

Sterilization of instruments and accessories is safely carried out by the ethylene oxide method available in most hospitals. Cold sterilization can also be done using a solution such as 2% glutaraldehyde. The instrument should soak for at least 20 min (1).

REFERENCES

1. Boyce WH Jr (1982): Laparoscopy. In: *Diseases of the Liver*, edited by L Schiff and ER Schiff, pp. 333–348. JB Lippincott Company, Philadelphia.
2. Beck K (1982): *Color Atlas of Laparoscopy*. WB Saunders Company, Philadelphia.

24 / Percutaneous Transhepatic Cholangiography

Sidney L. Levinson

Percutaneous transhepatic cholangiography (PTC) is a diagnostic modality useful in differentiating intrahepatic and extrahepatic causes of cholestasis or in localizing biliary tract obstruction. The study delineates changes in intrahepatic bile ducts and the common bile duct, and it is especially effective in identifying gallstones, parasites, and such space-occupying lesions as bifurcation tumors (1,2). PTC offers an alternative in evaluation of jaundice with incomplete ERCP, a Billroth II anastomosis, or in patients who cannot tolerate endoscopy (3).

When a mechanical obstruction of the biliary tract is suspected, PTC may be preferred over ERCP as the initial approach (3). PTC may also be preferred in patients with known dilated ducts, where the diagnostic yield approaches 100% (1,4,5). The high diagnostic yield with PTC in some centers among jaundiced patients with nondilated ducts makes the procedure a valuable first step in the evaluation of suspected biliary obstruction (2,5).

Indications

1. Diagnosis of obstructive jaundice.
2. Establishment of anatomic detail of intrahepatic and extrahepatic bile ducts.
3. Identification of stones, parasites, bifurcation tumors, and other space-occupying lesions.
4. Highlighting changes of biliary tree in pancreatic disease (e.g., chronic pancreatitis).

Contraindications

Absolute

1. Bleeding abnormalities (see Chapter 23, Peritoneoscopy).
2. Active sepsis, peritonitis, or cellulitis of abdominal wall.
3. Sensitivity to iodine contrast media.

Relative

1. High or continuous fever (some authors recommend use of antibiotics).
2. Moderate to severe anemia.
3. Recent pain of probable biliary tract origin.
4. Ascites.
5. Metastatic cancer involving the liver.

Preparation

Antibiotics

Antibiotics may be given prior to the procedure. Some authors recommend it for all patients (1,2,6), whereas others use antibiotics only if the patients are icteric or if there is a history of cholangitis (3). For patients without signs of active infection, ampicillin or cefoxitin, 4 g/day in divided doses can be used; chloramphenicol, 3 to 4 g/day, is an alternative, particularly in penicillin-sensitive patients. Tobramycin, 3 to 5 mg/kg/day in divided doses, may be added in instances of cholangitis or sepsis. Cefaperazone, a cephalosporin that is concentrated in bile, may be used as a single agent in divided doses totaling 4 g/day.

Coagulation Parameters

Check coagulation parameters and institute measures to correct abnormalities (vitamin K, cessation of aspirin several days to weeks prior to procedure, administration of plasma or various concentrates in patients with documented factor deficiencies).

Equipment

1. The Chiba needle. This is available commercially as a 22-gauge needle, 15 cm long, with an inner fitting stylet and a short 30° noncutting bevel. The inner diameter is 0.5 mm, and the outer diameter is 0.7 mm.
2. Fluoroscopy suite. Emergency facilities to manage dye reactions or other complications are needed in the unit.
3. Povidone iodine solution, injectable lidocaine, and sterile drapes for preparation of the needle stick site.
4. Renografin or other solutions (e.g., 60% meglumine isothalamate, 60% sodium meglumine diatrozoate) for use as contrast.
5. Intravenous diazepam. This may be used as premedication.

Procedure (1–7)

1. Place the patient supine on the fluoroscopy table; support the head with the patient's right arm.
2. Drape the lower right lateral chest wall and prepare with povidone iodine solution.
3. Select the area of puncture in the eighth or ninth intercostal space (based on liver size). This is just below the costophrenic angle, at or just anterior to the midaxillary line (10–13 cm off the table). The lateral approach provides a longer tract for tamponade of blood and bile.
4. Locally infiltrate the area with lidocaine.
5. Have the patient hold his breath at end of expiration and pass the needle, with stylet in place, horizontal to the table. *The pass is made under fluoroscopic control, aimed toward a point just to the left of the dome of the right diaphragm, avoiding the confluence of the main hepatic ducts* (Fig. 1). The border of the vertebral bodies is used as an endpoint for the pass; however, some authors do not rely on the often inconstant relationships of the liver, lung, and vertebrae (7).
6. Remove the stylet and attach a syringe filled with contrast.
7. With the patient resuming shallow respirations, withdraw the needle slowly, several millimeters at a time. Apply

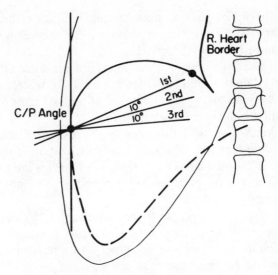

FIG. 1. Insertion of Chiba needle.

gentle pressure to the plunger while injecting 0.1 to 1.0 ml of contrast. The pattern of contrast seen on fluoroscopy will determine a successful injection. Slow hepatofugal flow in linear structures, which may be persistent, particularly with obstruction, denotes bile ducts (3,5). Other possible patterns include the following:

a. An indistinct blush usually denotes liver parenchyma.
b. Serpiginous thin vessels flowing to the liver hilum are lymph vessels.
c. A stellate network of channels carrying contrast rapidly to the liver hilum and on to the right atrium denotes blood vessels.

8. Fill the ducts with a minimum of contrast. Aspiration of bile is usually not necessary. However, if dilated ducts are encountered, bile is removed in 30- to 100-cc amounts, and contrast is given cubic centimeter for cubic centimeter. Take care to avoid overdistension of the ducts. Sepsis is more likely to occur with dilated ducts containing bile under pressure. Instill no more than 5 cc per pass if no duct is found.

9. If the initial pass is unsuccessful, reposition the needle successively in 10° increments caudally, then slightly more anteriorly or posteriorly (Fig. 1).

10. Most authors conclude that ducts are not dilated if no enlarged duct is found after six passes (1–4), whereas others will try up to 15 passes because of the low risks for morbidity with successive passes (5,7).

11. Take X-rays with fluoroscopy and overhead shots, including semierect shots for best visualization of the distal ducts. Normal ducts range from 3 to 7 mm for intrahepatic, 4 to 8 mm for common hepatic, and 5 to 11 mm for the common bile duct.

12. If nondilated ducts are found, inject up to 15 cc contrast. More may be injected if the gallbladder is present.

13. Aspirate at the end of the procedure. Decompression is particularly important with dilated ducts.

14. Send specimens for culture and cytologic study.

Interpretation (5)

Experience with PTC has shed light on specific fluoroscopic patterns that might affect interpretation of the procedure. When properly performed, PTC can allow visualization of 95% to 100% of dilated biliary ducts. Nondilated ducts are visualized in 60% to 95% of cases.

1. A linear tract of contrast is created on withdrawal of the needle during a pass. This may act as a conduit for preferential flow of contrast to venous structures that were already hit and divert contrast from smaller biliary radicles hit later.

2. The lymphatic pattern, serpiginous blood vessels, may be confused with sclerosing biliary radicles, although the course is different.

3. Some radicles may be adequate for filling the duct system and yet not be seen on fluoroscopy. It is important to scan carefully with fluoroscopy over the area of the common duct after each pass to look for filling.

4. Stagnant bile in the distal ducts can cause false proximal localization of the site of obstruction or may cause pseu-

dodefects caused by poor admixture of contrast. This problem may be solved with delayed upright and/or prone films.
5. Dissection of dye through the adventitia of large vessels can be identified by slow flow in a broad pattern.

Postprocedure

1. Obtain a chest X-ray to rule out pneumothorax.
2. Monitor vital signs and observe the patient for signs of hemorrhage, peritonitis, or sepsis.
3. Use antibiotics (see Preparation, Antibiotics) if there are dilated ducts with complete obstruction or if signs of sepsis or cholangitis develop.
4. A diagnosis of high-grade obstruction in conjunction with signs of complications usually requires emergency surgery.
5. An alternative approach to surgery for high-grade biliary tract obstruction is the performance of percutaneous catheter drainage. This procedure is performed by radiologists/angiographers and is beyond the scope of this manual.

Complications (1–8)

Major complications are due to dilatation of ducts, not the number of passes (7). The incidence of complications increases if catheter drainage is performed (8).

Major

1. Fever and hypotension (2%).
2. Cholangitis with sepsis (2). Bacteremia usually occurs with gallstones, bile duct cancer, or pancreatic cancer.
3. Peritonitis (1–2%), with bile leakage in up to 5% in patients with obstruction (8).
4. Bleeding (1–2%). A patient's inability to hold his breath may increase the risk of bleeding.
5. Bile embolism, with portal vein branch puncture (<1%).
6. Gallbladder puncture (<1%).

Minor (15% Incidence)

1. Subcapsular hematoma.
2. Capsular laceration.

3. Pneumothorax.
4. Transient but severe epigastric pain. This pain, caused by parenchymal extravasation, correlates with the number of passes. Local guarding may be found, and nausea and hypotension may develop, all clearing within 30 min with no sequellae.

REFERENCES

1. Okuda K, Tanikawa K, Emura T, et al (1974): Nonsurgical, percutaneous transhepatic cholangiography—diagnostic significance in medical problems of the liver. *Am J Dig Dis* 19:21–36.
2. Pereiras R Jr, Chiprut RO, Greenwald RA, Schiff E (1977): Percutaneous transhepatic cholangiography with the "skinny" needle. A rapid, simple, and accurate method in the diagnosis of cholestasis. *Ann Int Med* 86:562–568.
3. Ferrucci JT Jr, Wittenberg J, Sarno RA, Dreyfuss JR (1976): Fine needle transhepatic cholangiography: a new approach to obstructive jaundice. *Am J Radiol* 127:403–407.
4. Redeker AG, Karvountzis GG, Richman RH, Horisawa M (1975): Percutaneous transhepatic cholangiography. An improved technique. *JAMA* 231:386–387.
5. Ferrucci JT Jr, Wittenberg J (1977): Refinements in Chiba needle transhepatic cholangiography. *Am J Radiol* 129:11–16.
6. Elias E, Hamlyn AN, Jain S, et al (1976): A randomized trial of PTC with the Chiba needle versus ERC for bile duct visualization in jaundice. *Gastroenterology* 71:439–443.
7. Jaques PF, Mauro MA, Scatliff JH (1980): The failed transhepatic cholangiogram. *Radiology* 134:33–35.
8. Voegeli DR, Crummy AB, Weese JL (1985): Percutaneous transhepatic cholangiography, drainage, and biopsy in patients with malignant biliary obstruction. An alternative to surgery. *Am J Surg* 150:243–247.

25 / Dilatation of the Esophagus: Mercury-Filled Bougies (Hurst-Maloney)

Eugene M. Bozymski

Esophageal stricture is a severe complication of gastroesophageal reflux and once established is difficult to manage in an entirely satisfactory manner. One of the mainstays in treating such strictures, as well as other entities that obliterate the esophageal lumen, is periodic dilatation. The oldest, least expensive, and still frequently used method is the use of mercury-filled bougies of graded sizes. Two main types are available: the blunt rounded Hurst dilators and the tapered Maloney dilators (Fig. 1).

Indications

1. Peptic esophageal strictures.
2. Caustic strictures.
3. Radiation-induced strictures.
4. Palliation for esophageal carcinoma.
5. Upper esophageal webs.
6. Lower esophageal rings.
7. Occasionally for diffuse esophageal spasm.

Contraindications

1. Significant bleeding diathesis.
2. Recent (within 10 to 14 days) esophageal biopsies, particularly those obtained with a Rubin-Quinton multipurpose suction biopsy tube.

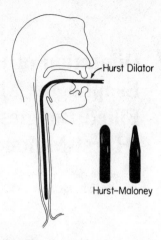

FIG. 1. Hurst dilator being passed through esophageal stricture.

3. Impacted bolus.
4. Lack of patient cooperation.
5. Recent myocardial infarction.
6. Esophageal diverticulum.
7. Severe cervical arthritis.

Preparation

1. Obtain prior radiologic and/or endoscopic evaluation of the upper gastrointestinal tract.
2. If the stricture is so severe that caloric intake has been markedly impaired, hospitalize the patients and perform the dilatations over several days.
3. Nothing by mouth for 8 hr.
4. Obtain informed, written consent.
5. Anesthetize the pharynx with a topical agent, such as cetacaine or hurricaine.
6. Very *infrequently,* the patient may need preprocedure sedation with midazolam or meperidine.
7. If the patient has a prosthetic valve in place, one should follow the recommendations of the American Heart Association with respect to antibiotic therapy (see Chapters 12 and 15).

Equipment

1. Hurst and Maloney dilators.
2. Gloves, basin, gowns, and towels.
3. Lubricant.
4. Fluoroscopic equipment should be available, since confirmation of dilator position is occasionally necessary.

Procedure

1. The Hurst dilator with its blunt end should be the initial bougie used for most strictures of the esophagus. Maloney dilators with their tapered end are often used for longer strictures because the tapered end serves as a lumen finder.
2. Start with the size most appropriate, based on the previous endoscopic examination or a prior dilatation. For example, if the stricture was judged to be 6 mm in transverse diameter on endoscopic exam, an 18 French Hurst bougie should be used as the initial dilator (1 mm is roughly equivalent to 3 French). If the patient was dilated to 30 French 1 week earlier, it would be appropriate to start the subsequent dilatation with the same-size bougie.
3. Seat the patient lower than the operator and place the dilator in the posterior pharynx, resting it on the cricopharyngeus.
4. Ask the patient to swallow.
5. Pass the tube (while the nurse assists) by keeping the weighted column of mercury above the patient's head.
6. If passage through the stricture is difficult, it often helps to place the volar surface of the index and middle fingers of the left hand against the hard palate to anchor the bougie in place while exerting mild pressure with the right hand on the bougie. Most often a "pop" or a "give" can be felt as the stricture is passed. Also, greater resistance is noted when pulling the dilator back through the stricture.
7. Dilatations are carried out with three to four dilators, depending on the ease of the procedure and patient tolerance. Stop the dilatation at the point where blood is noted on the dilator or if the patient complains of severe pain.

8. Redilate the stricture within a few days, starting with the size of the last dilator from the previous dilatation. If it will not pass, drop back a size or two and work up again.

9. With short strictures, larger dilators may at times pass more easily, whereas smaller dilators will be too flimsy. Proceed with caution.

10. Fluoroscopic confirmation is necessary when there is a question as to whether the bougie is passing through the stricture. At times, the bougie may simply curl in the esophagus or push the esophagus ahead and not pass the stricture.

11. Endoscopic biopsies are usually obtained 10 to 14 days prior to the first dilatation to exclude a neoplastic stricture; however, when the stricture precludes adequate nutritional intake, dilatation should be performed. Brush cytologies should be obtained prior to the procedure. Once the stricture is dilated sufficiently to allow passage of the endoscope, complete examination of the esophagus along with biopsies can be accomplished.

12. With dilatation of a lower esophageal ring (Schatzki's ring), two methods have been recommended. One approach is to use graded French Hurst dilators and progress from 32 to 36 to 42 or 40 to 44 to 48. This allows one to stretch as well as rupture the mucosal ring. The other approach is to begin dilatation with one large (44–50 French) bougie.

Postprocedure

1. Most often, the procedures described in this chapter are done on an outpatient basis. The physician must advise the patient to notify him or her immediately if there is chest or back pain, fever, regurgitation, or vomiting of blood.

2. The patient should take nothing by mouth until the anesthetic agent wears off. This can be tested by having the patient attempt to swallow small quantities of water 1 hr after the procedure has been completed.

3. Administer antacids or sucralfate for 4 to 5 days following the procedure.

Complications

1. Esophageal perforation (<0.01%).
2. Hemorrhage (<0.04%).
3. Aspiration.
4. Bacteremia.

REFERENCES

1. Rosenow EC (1974): Techniques of esophageal dilatation. In: *The Esophagus,* edited by WS Payne and AM Olsen, pp. 55–64. Lea and Febiger, Philadelphia.
2. Patterson DJ, Graham DY, Smith JL, Schwartz JT, Alpert E, Lanza FL, Cain GD (1983): Natural history of benign esophageal stricture treated by dilatation. *Gastroenterology* 85:346–350.
3. Welsh JD, Griffiths WJ, McKee J, Wilkinson D, Flournoy DJ, Mohr JA (1983): Bacteremia associated with esophageal dilatation. *J Clin Gastroenterol* 5:109–112.
4. Tulman AB, Boyce HW Jr (1981): Complications of esophageal dilation and guidelines for their prevention. *Gastrointest Endosc* 27:229–234.

26 / Dilatation of the Esophagus: Wire-Guided Bougies (Eder-Puestow and Savary-Gilliard Bougies)

Eugene M. Bozymski

Dilatation of very narrow strictures can be carried out by passing bougies of various sizes over previously passed guide wires. A wire with a flexible spring tip can be substituted for the guide wire. This latter system represents the Eder-Puestow wire-guide method of dilating the esophagus and is very useful for initiating dilatation of tight strictures through which a mercury-filled bougie will not pass. The Eder-Puestow system includes a flexible wire with a coiled spring tip (which can be passed through the biopsy channel of an endoscope), a set of olive dilators of various calibers, and flexible steel pusher rod to which the various dilators can be screwed. The entire assembly then can be passed over the previously passed flexible wire, which serves as a guide wire. The obvious advantage to such a system is that the dilating olive must follow the wire and cannot stray within the lumen, thus decreasing the chance of perforation.

Savary-Gilliard dilators are centrally drilled tapered dilators that can be passed over a previously placed guide wire. Otherwise, the technique is much the same as with Hurst-Maloney dilators (see Chapter 25). With the advantage that these dilators are able to follow the guide wire through the lumen, the Savary-

Gilliard system appears to be easier and safer than the Eder-Puestow dilators.

We are also now using a wide array of polyethylene balloon (Gruentzig) dilators, passed directly through the biopsy channel of the endoscope or over an endoscopically placed tiny flexible .035 guide wire, in the management of esophageal strictures, and this technique is discussed in Chapter 28. The choice of which dilator to use in the management of esophageal strictures is still to be determined.

Indications

Puestow dilatation is used for strictures that are too small to be dilated with mercury-filled bougies. [See also Hurst-Maloney dilatation (Chapter 25).]

Contraindications

1. See Hurst-Maloney dilatation (Chapter 25).
2. Esophageal ulcer.

Preparation

1. Check the hematocrit, platelet count, PT, and PTT.
2. Review cervical spine films (if previously obtained) for arthritis.
3. Obtain written, informed consent.
4. Administer topical anesthetic to pharynx.
5. Start an i.v. for administration of atropine and diazepam, midazolam, or meperidine as necessary.

Equipment

1. Endoscope (recommended for first dilatation).
2. Puestow guide wire with olive dilators of varying size and flexible rod.
3. Fluoroscope.
4. Lubricant and gloves.

Procedure

1. Endoscope the patient prior to the first dilatation. This will allow observation of any anatomic esophageal variation, such as the presence of pseudodiverticula or true diverticula, as well as any tortuosity or eccentrically located strictures. If an ulcer is identified, dilatation should be postponed until an antireflux program reduces the inflammation.

2. During direct observation at endoscopy, place the guide wire through the stricture well into the stomach. Pull the endoscope out 5 cm at a time while advancing the wire 5 cm so that the wire tip will remain in position in the stomach.

3. On removal of the endoscope, check the wire position fluoroscopically to make certain that the tip remains in the stomach, well below the stricture.

4. Oral passage of the guide wire without endoscopy may be performed in patients undergoing repeated dilatation. This can be accomplished by having the patient swallow a shortened slit nasogastric or small tube of any type and advancing the guide wire through it. The position of the wire in the stomach must be confirmed by fluoroscopy.

5. Begin the dilatation by passing the smallest available olive over the wire.

6. Gently advance the olive into the body of the esophagus through the posterior pharynx and cricopharyngeus. Advance the Puestow rod over the guide wire for short distances at a time, maintaining good control by holding the Puestow rod close to the patient's mouth and advancing slowly (Fig. 1).

7. As the stricture is reached, increased resistance is noted and more pressure may be needed to pass through the stricture.

8. Successful passage of the dilator through the stricture should be confirmed fluoroscopically.

9. After the dilator has passed the stricture and one begins to pull it back, the resistance of the stricture will again be felt as the dilator passes through it.

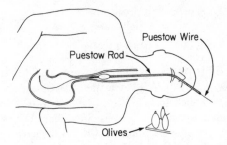

FIG. 1. Puestow wire in place with flexible tip in the stomach. The dilating olive is advanced through the stricture with the Puestow rod.

10. Retrieve the dilator by pulling it back over the guide wire in short, 2- to 5-cm segments.
11. Continue with three to four progressive dilators or until blood is noted on the dilator, whereupon the procedure is terminated.
12. Subsequent Puestow dilatations can be performed by passing the wire through the mouth into the stomach under fluoroscopic control. Endoscopic placement is not necessary prior to every Puestow dilatation unless one encounters problems. However, fluoroscopic confirmation of the wire placement is always necessary prior to undertaking a Puestow dilatation.

Postprocedure

1. See Chapter 25.
2. Monitor vital signs.
3. Elevate the head of the bed.
4. Clear liquids for 24 hr: then if clinically stable, soft diet for 2 days; then routine diet.
5. Antacids 30 cc between meals and at bedtime for 5 days. Sucralfate 1 gm q.i.d. for 5 days is an alternative.

Complications

1. Esophageal perforation (~0.3%).
2. Hemorrhage (<0.1%).
3. Aspiration.

4. Bacteremia.

REFERENCES

1. Rosenow EC (1974): Techniques of esophageal dilatation. In: *The Esophagus,* edited by WS Payne and AM Olsen, pp. 55–64. Lea and Febiger, Philadelphia.
2. Mandelstam P, Sugawa C, Silvis SE, Nebel OT, Rogers BHG (1976): Complications associated with esophagogastroduodenoscopy and with esophageal dilatation. *Gastrointest Endos* 23:16–19.
3. Monnier P, Hsieh V, Savary M (1985): Endoscopic treatment of esophageal stenosis using Savary-Gilliard bougies: technical innovations. *Acta Endos* 15:1–5.

27 / Dilatation of the Esophagus: Pneumatic (Brown-McHardy)

Eugene M. Bozymski

Pneumatic dilatation of the esophagus is one of the major modalities used in the treatment of achalasia. In our department, it is preferred in most instances over surgical myotomy (Heller procedure). The main feature of pneumatic dilatation is that it is a forceful dilatation compared to passive dilatation accomplished by passing a mercury-filled bougie. We use the Brown-McHardy dilator, which consists of a cloth bag of fixed diameter covered by a rubber sheath near the end of a mercury-filled bougie. Air is pumped into this bag and the pressure (pounds per square inch) monitored on a manometer (Fig. 1). The intended purpose of this forceful dilatation is to decrease the resistance at the lower esophageal sphincter and to allow the esophagus to empty more readily.

A variety of other dilators are available for use in treating the patient with achalasia. These include those that can be attached to an endoscope or passed directly over a flexible guide wire. These may be very useful in the patient with a "sigmoid" esophagus.

Indications

1. Achalasia.
2. Certain patients with diffuse esophageal spasm with hypertensive sphincter.

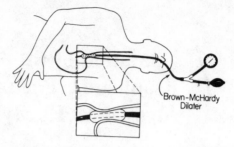

FIG. 1. The pneumatic dilator in place at the lower esophageal sphincter (monitored fluoroscopically).

Contraindications

Absolute

1. Significant bleeding dyscrasia.
2. Esophageal varices.
3. No prior endoscopy.
4. Epiphrenic diverticulum.
5. Recent esophageal mucosal biopsy in the sphincteric area.
6. No prior manometry.

Relative (depends on the clinical situation): Esophagitis (stasis)

Preparation

1. Obtain informed, written consent.
2. Spray the pharynx with a topical anesthetic.
3. Start an i.v. for administration of atropine and midazolam or diazepam.

Equipment

1. Endoscope.
2. Gastric lavage tube.
3. Brown-McHardy dilator.
4. Fluoroscope.
5. Gloves and lubricant.

Procedure

1. If there is any debris in the esophagus, empty it with a large-bore gastric lavage tube.
2. Perform upper endoscopy to exclude lesions, such as carcinoma of the fundus presenting as "secondary achalasia" and other diseases of the distal esophagus.
3. Instruct the patient to report with a hand signal when severe chest pain occurs during the dilatation.
4. Pass the Brown-McHardy dilator as one would pass a large, mercury-filled bougie.
5. Position the dilator so that the bag straddles the high-pressure zone. Confirm this fluoroscopically. If positioned too low, the bag is propelled into the stomach with insufflation. If positioned too high, it will retract into the esophagus. When the bag is positioned properly, an hourglass effect is observed (Fig. 2a).
6. Insufflate the bag under fluoroscopic control while the assistant monitors the pressure on the manometer. We have adopted a conservative policy for pneumatic dilatation and would prefer having the patient come back for another dilatation rather than performing the initial procedure too vigorously. In our institution, we use fluoroscopic control and patient response to determine how long to leave the bag blown up. In general, most dilatations require pressures of 9 to 12 pounds per square inch for 5 to 10 sec to be effective; however, the fluoroscopic appearance and the presence of pain should be guidelines for the extent of dilatation rather than any absolute time or pressure. There are many different methods of forceful dilatation, and it is not known whether the diameter of the bag, the filling pres-

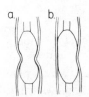

FIG. 2. a: Note the hourglass appearance of the balloon in the lower esophageal sphincter. **b**: The balloon has now expanded on one side.

sure of the bag, or the duration of the dilatation is most important in obtaining a good result.

7. Ideally, one of the sides of the hourglass should straighten (Fig. 2b).
8. When the bag straightens or the patient develops severe pain, rapidly deflate the bag and remove the dilator. Most often, small amounts of blood will be noted on the dilating bag following dilatation.

Postprocedure

1. Observe the patient in the hospital overnight following dilatation.
2. Instruct the patient to inform you of continuing chest pain, back pain, or pain elsewhere.
3. Monitor vital signs.
4. Elevate the head of the bed.
5. Chest X-ray 5 to 6 hr postprocedure.
6. A Gastrografin swallow may be obtained the following morning to study esophageal emptying; however, some physicians recommend an immediate postdilatation esophagogram to exclude an esophageal perforation.
7. Hematocrit the following morning.
8. Clear liquids for 24 hr and if clinically stable, soft diet for 2 days, then regular diet.
9. Antacids 30 cc 1 hr p.c. and h.s. for 5 days. Sucralfate has been used in a similar fashion.

Complications

Esophageal Perforation

The dreaded complication of any esophageal dilatation is esophageal perforation (0.6–2.5%) (1,2). This complication should be highly suspect if chest pain persists for more than 15 min following the dilatation or if it involves the back or the left side. The onset of fever is another ominous feature. Should perforation be suspected, the patient should be taken to the radiology department and a chest X-ray obtained, which may show a left pleural effusion or mediastinal air. Even if normal, the patient should have a Gastrografin swallow to check for a leak. If none is found, barium then should be substituted and the exam repeated. It is important to turn the patient in all positions so that if a leak is present, it will be detected. Once a leak is demonstrated, thoracic surgical consultation should be sought, and most often, surgery is indicated if the leak is discovered early. Others have reported the effective use of antibiotics and parenteral feeding, along with drainage of pleural effusions until the tear closes.

Other Complications

1. Hemorrhage, <1% to 2%.
2. Aspiration.

REFERENCES

1. Vantrappen G, Janssens J, Hellemans J, Coremans G (1979): Achalasia, 1 diffuse esophageal spasm and related motility disorders. *Gastroenterology* 76:450–457.
2. Vantrappen G, Hellemans J (1980): Treatment of achalasia and related motility disorders. *Gastroenterology* 79:144–154.
3. Rosenow EC (1974): Techniques of esophageal dilatation. In: *The Esophagus,* edited by WS Payne and AM Olsen, pp. 55–64. Lea and Febiger, Philadelphia.
4. Jacobs JB, Cohen NL, Mattel S (1983): Pneumatic dilatation as the primary treatment for achalasia. *Ann Otol Rhinol Laryngol* 92:353–356.
5. Witzel L (1981): Treatment of achalasia with a pneumatic dilator attached to a gastroscope. *Endoscopy* 13:176–177.

28 / Balloon Dilatation of Strictures (Gruentzig)

William D. Heizer

Most esophageal strictures may be easily and safely dilated with mercury-filled bougies or Eder-Puestow dilators. Use of low-compliance balloons for dilatation of strictures in the gastrointestinal tract is a recent innovation that appears to offer some advantages. First, compared to the established methods, balloon dilatation may be safer because it applies only radial pressure to the narrowed area (1–3), although a recent retrospective survey did not confirm increased safety (4). Second, some esophageal strictures that are too narrow or complex for treatment with mercury-filled or Eder-Puestow dilators can be managed with balloon dilatation (5). Third, strictures in the stomach, duodenum, colon, biliary tract, and pancreatic duct that are not amenable to treatment by the older methods have been successfully dilated by balloon catheters (6–9).

In spite of the apparent advantages of balloon dilatation, it should be noted that the safety, effectiveness, and comfort of the various dilatation methods have not been directly compared. Furthermore, current techniques for dilatation with balloon catheters require either endoscopy or fluoroscopy, with each dilatation making the balloon method more expensive and time-consuming than use of mercury-filled dilators for treatment of known esophageal strictures.

Few technical aspects of balloon dilatation have been firmly established. Consequently, details, such as balloon sizes, number of balloon sizes for each dilatation, pressure, and duration of pressure, are largely matters of personal choice.

Indications

Dilatation of benign or malignant strictures of the gastrointestinal tract.

Contraindications

Absolute Contraindications

1. Uncooperative patient.
2. Perforation, ulcer, recent biopsy, or severe inflammation at or near the stricture site.

Relative Contraindication

Uncorrectable coagulation disorder.

Preparation

1. Patient's stomach should be empty.
2. Consent form signed.
3. Test balloon with air for leaks or defects.
4. Fill a syringe with one part water-soluble contrast solution and three parts water. Be sure that volume of dilute contrast is sufficient to distend fully the largest balloon that will be used.
5. Topical anesthesia of pharynx with lidocaine or Cetacaine.
6. Intravenous diazepam and meperidine as required.

Equipment

1. Balloon dilators in sizes from 6 mm in diameter (19 French) to 19 mm in diameter (60 French). Balloon catheters up to 54 French, which can pass through the 2.8-mm endoscope channel.
2. Flexible wire guide of appropriate diameter and length.
3. Endoscope or fluoroscope, depending on the method to be used.
4. Mouth suction.

Procedure for Esophageal Dilatation

Insert Wire Guide

If endoscopy is not required, pass the wire guide through the esophageal stricture well into the stomach using fluoroscopic guidance. Alternatively, pass the wire through the stricture under direct vision via the channel of an endoscope. Use the endoscope to measure the distance from the incisor teeth to the stricture for later reference. Maintain the wire in place and remove the endoscope by withdrawing the endoscope a few centimeters at a time while the wire is advanced at the same rate.

Insert Balloon Catheter

We generally use a single large-diameter balloon (36–60 French) and judge dilatation by fluoroscopy and/or the degree of patient discomfort rather than using a series of balloons of increasing diameter. If endoscopy has been done, use the incisor-to-stricture measurement to mark the balloon catheter so that when the mark is at the incisor tip, the balloon will straddle the stricture.

Remove all air or fluid from the balloon to be used and lubricate the balloon. Advance the balloon catheter over the wire into the stomach and, at the same time, avoid withdrawing the tip of the wire from the stomach or advancing it excessively.

Dilate Stricture

If fluoroscopy is to be used, instill a few milliliters of the diluted contrast into the balloon to visualize it. Once it has been localized in the stomach, instill more contrast and withdraw the loosely filled balloon until it straddles the stricture, as indicated by a waist in the midportion of the balloon (Fig. 1A). Inflate the balloon and keep steady, firm pressure on the syringe for 15 to 120 sec. Observe the balloon with short bursts of fluoroscopy to note the increase in diameter of the stricture (i.e., loss of the waist, Fig. 1B). The amount and duration of pressure should be determined by the appearance of the waist, patient discomfort, and previous experience with the particular

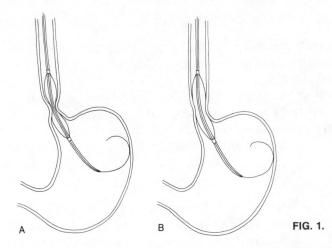

A   B   FIG. 1.

patient. Some physicians prefer a pressure gauge in the system to avoid exceeding balloon pressure limits. A gauge is especially important when fluoroscopy is not used for observation during dilatation. We do not exceed a pressure of 45 lb/in^2.

The technique of "blind retrograde balloon dilatation" avoids the use of fluoroscopy. Fully inflate the balloon in the stomach and withdraw until resistance from the stricture is encountered. Then, partially deflate the balloon, withdraw 3 cm, and reinflate. Deflate, withdraw another 3 cm, and reinflate. Repeat this process two to three times more to assure dilatation of the stricture. The previously applied mark on the balloon catheter serves to confirm proper location of the balloon. Finally, push the deflated balloon back into the stomach, reinflate fully, and withdraw through the strictured area to judge effectiveness of the dilatation. When this method is used, begin with a small-diameter balloon and advance by two to four balloon sizes at each dilatation session.

Balloon catheters can be passed through the endoscope channel or over a wire passed beside the endoscope. Dilatation can then be carried out under direct vision. This technique is particularly useful for strictures in the stomach, duodenum, and colon.

Postprocedure

1. Instruct the patient not to eat or drink anything until the topical anesthetic has worn off.
2. Liquid diet for 12 hr.
3. Instruct the patient what to do if gastrointestinal bleeding or severe chest pain or abdominal pain should occur.
4. Give antiacid and antireflux treatment if the stricture is acid peptic in origin.

Complications

The true incidence of complications is unknown. A recent survey uncovered 11 hemorrhages and two perforations in 617 balloon dilatations of the esophagus, a 2.1% complication rate (4). There were four perforations and one hemorrhage among 545 gastric dilatations (0.9%) and three perforations and two hemorrhages following 64 colon dilatations (7.8%). Many of these complications were attributed to the sharp tip of the balloon catheter, and softer tipped catheters are now available. Other potential complications include aspiration, allergic reactions, bacteremia, and radiation damage. Cholangitis and pancreatitis appear to occur with rather high frequency following balloon dilatations of biliary and pancreatic duct strictures (4).

REFERENCES

1. Graham DY (1985): Dilatation for the management of benign and malignant strictures of the esophagus. In: *Therapeutic Gastrointestinal Endoscopy,* edited by Stephen E Silvis, pp 1–30. Igaku-Shoin, New York.
2. Graham DY, Smith JL (1985): Balloon dilatation of benign and malignant esophageal strictures: blind retrograde balloon dilatation. *Gastrointest Endosc* 31:171–174.
3. Starck E, Paolucci V, Herzer M, Crummy AB (1984): Esophageal stenosis: treatment with balloon catheters. *Radiology* 953:637–640.
4. Kozarek RA (1986): Hydrostatic balloon dilatation of gastrointestinal stenoses: a national survey. *Gastrointest Endosc* 32:15–18.
5. London RL, Trotman BW, DiMarino AJ, Oleaga JA, Freiman DB,

Ring EJ, Rosato EF (1981): Dilatation of severe esophageal strictures by an inflatable balloon catheter. *Gastroenterology* 80:173–175.

6. Eckhauser FE, Knol JA, Strodel JWE, Cho K (1984): Hydrostatic balloon dilatation for stomal stenosis after gastric partitioning. *Surg Gastroenterol* 3:43–50.

7. Hutson DG, Russell E, Schiff E, Levi JJ, Jeffers L, Zeppa R (1984): Balloon dilatation of biliary strictures through a choledochojejunocutaneous fistula. *Ann Surg* 199:637–647.

8. Foutch PG, Sivak MV (1985): Therapeutic endoscopic balloon dilatation of the extrahepatic ducts. *Am J Gastroenterol* 80:575–580.

9. Guelrud M, Siegel JH (1984): Hypertensive pancreatic duct sphincter as a cause of pancreatitis: successful treatment with hydrostatic balloon dilatation. *Dig Dis Sci* 39:225–231.

29 / Endoscopic Sclerosis of Esophageal Varices

Eugene M. Bozymski

Bleeding from esophageal varices is one of the most difficult problems confronting gastroenterologists and surgeons. A wide variety of therapeutic manuvers have been developed to control the bleeding. Currently, one way to control hemorrhage on a long-term basis is the use of decompressive portal systemic shunt surgery; however, many patients, because of co-existing medical problems (usually decompensated liver disease) or because of technical problems, are not suitable shunt candidates. It is this group of patients that led Terblanche to reintroduce endoscopic sclerosis of varices, which had been practiced many years earlier. Sclerotherapy has been shown to be effective in controlling bleeding in the acute situation and also is effective in the long-term management of this type of patient.

Indications

1. To stop acute hemorrhage from esophageal varices.
2. To ablate esophageal varices causing recurrent hemorrhage.
3. Temporizing measure to control bleeding in patients with poor hepatic reserve in anticipation of shunt surgery, if condition improves.
4. Patients with variceal hemorrhage who are not operative candidates.

Contraindications

1. Uncooperative patient.
2. More than mildly abnormal clotting factors.

Preparation

1. Patient should have been seen by Vascular Surgery Service.
2. Obtain written, informed consent.
3. Blood sample in blood bank.
4. Establish a venous access.
5. Meperidine, diazepam or midazolam, atropine, and glucagon should be available.

Equipment

1. If the potential for balloon tamponade is thought necessary, cut the end off a condom and make it into a simple sheath. Place it over the distal part of the endoscope and double it back over itself. Fix it at its distal end by a rubber band. Slide a polyethylene tube into the condom at its proximal end, which is also fixed by rubber bands. Tape the small polyethylene tube along the shaft of the endoscope. Then, attach a syringe to this catheter and blow air into the balloon for inflation purposes. Air can be deflated from the balloon by aspiration. We no longer routinely use the balloon modification, but use a twin-channel gastroscope and direct puncture of the varix followed by injection.
2. Injector (23 ga, 4-mm needle). A variety of disposable injectors are also available from a number of suppliers. The injector should be tested for patency prior to use.
3. Two to three 10-cc syringes filled with 5% sodium morrhuate.
4. Safety goggles.
5. Teaching attachment or TV monitor.
6. Gloves and lubricant.

Procedure

1. Anesthetize the patient's pharynx with topical anesthetic.
2. Premedicate the patient with 0.5 mg atropine, along with meperidine and midazolam as needed.
3. Pass the gastroscope.

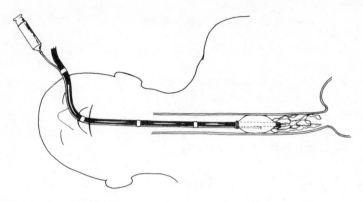

FIG. 1. Sclerotherapy of esophageal varices.

4. Inspect the esophagus, stomach, and duodenum for other possible sources of bleeding.
5. Identify the esophageal varices and note their extent.
6. The physician and assistants must put protective safety goggles in place and place a towel over the patient's eyes to protect against accidental spraying of sclerosing agent.
7. Reposition the scope to identify the varices just above the esophagogastric junction.
8. Pass the injector until it is visualized in the lumen over the varix and impale it. On command, the assistant injects 1 to 3 cc sodium morrhuate (Fig. 1).
9. Remove the needle and observe the varix for excessive bleeding.
10. Sequentially inject all varices present at that level. Advance the gastroscope into the stomach and aspirate air.
11. Move the scope cephalad 4 to 5 cm and repeat the procedure.
12. Again withdraw the endoscope approximately 4 cm and repeat the injection.
13. If a specific vein is to be injected at multiple sites, use smaller volumes (0.5–1.5 cc).
14. Remove the air from the stomach and remove the scope.
15. Other helpful hints:

   a. Do not inject greater than a total of approximately 20 to 30 cc sodium morrhuate during one procedure.

b. Expect to see either blanching or discoloration of the vein with some injections.

c. If a bleb begins to form at the injection site, stop—it may be too superficial.

d. If a bleeding point is identified on a varix, inject the varix below this point. If this is not possible due to excess blood, inject above or to the side of the bleeding point and then below. Some injections intended to be intravariceal will be paravariceal.

e. Some patients may experience pain at the time of injection.

f. Intravenous glucagon may be helpful in decreasing esophageal motility.

g. Some physicians prefer to do paravariceal injections. This technique involves injecting smaller volumes of sclerosant (0.5–1 cc per injection) *between* the varices at the level of the gastroesophageal junction. In theory, this technique leads to a fibrous band in the distal esophagus that prevents bleeding but does not obliterate the varices. In practice, some paravariceal injections will be intravariceal and vice versa.

16. The sclerotherapy may be repeated in 4 to 5 days and then again in a few weeks. Further sclerotherapy is then planned as needed.

17. If the balloon modification is used, follow these procedures:

a. When the varix to be injected is chosen, blow up the balloon with approximately 25 cc air.

b. Inject the varix and deflate the balloon.

c. If bleeding persists after injection, advance the scope a few centimeters so that the balloon portion is over the puncture site and inflate the balloon for 4 min. This usually controls the bleeding. If it persists, infuse i.v. vasopressin. Proceed with further injections as needed.

Postprocedure

1. Monitor vital signs.
2. Observe for any further signs of gastrointestinal blood loss.

3. When the patient's normal pharyngeal function has returned, clear liquid diet is permitted and continued for 24 hr.
4. Bed rest until the following morning.
5. Antacid 30 cc q. 1 hr while awake for the remainder of the day and then five to six times a day for the next 5 days. A sucralfate slurry can be used—1 g q.i.d.—in a similar fashion.
6. Liquid cimetidine 600 mg p.o. q. 12 hr for the next 5 days.
7. Hematocrit 6 hr postprocedure and again the following morning.

Complications

1. Hemorrhage from tearing the varix with the needle.
2. Ulceration of the esophagus at injection sites.
3. Postprocedure fever.
4. Perforation.
5. Pleural effusion.
6. Esophageal stricture.
7. Retrosternal pain may persist for a few days.

REFERENCES

1. Terblanche J (1985): A review of injection sclerotherapy—the Cape Town experience. *Jpn J Surg* 15:103–111.
2. VanHootegem P, Rutgeerts P, Fevery J, Broeckaert L, deGroote J, Vantrappen G (1984): Sclerotherapy of oesophageal varices after variceal haemorrhage. *Endoscopy* 16:95–97.
3. Endoscopic sclerotherapy for esophageal varices. Health and Public Policy Committee, American College of Physicians. (1984): *Ann Intern Med* 100:608–610.
4. Sivak MV Jr (1985): Sclerotherapy for esophageal varices. In: *Therapeutic Gastrointestinal Endoscopy*, edited by S. E. Silvis, pp. 31–66. Igaku Shoin, New York.
5. Fleig WE, Stange EF, Ruettenauer K, Ditschuneit H (1983): Emergency endoscopic sclerotherapy for bleeding esophageal varices: a prospective study in patients not responding to balloon tamponade. *Gastrointest Endosc* 29:8–14.
6. The Copenhagen Esophageal Varices Sclerotherapy Project. (1984): Sclerotherapy after first variceal hemorrhage in cirrhosis: a randomized multicenter trial. *N Engl J Med* 311:1594–1600.

7. Cello JP, Grendell JH, Crass RA, Trunkey DD, Cobb EE, Heilbron DC (1984): Endoscopic sclerotherapy portacaval shunt in patients with severe cirrhosis and variceal hemorrhage. *N Engl J Med* 311:1589–1594.

8. Paquet KJ (1982): Prophylactic endoscopic sclerosing treatment of the esophageal wall in varices—a prospective controlled randomized trial. *Endoscopy* 14:4–5.

30 / Percutaneous Endoscopic Gastrostomy

Eugene M. Bozymski

There are many patients in whom long-term enteral nutritional support is necessary. Patients with strokes or head and neck tumors that interfere with normal swallowing function previously have required a surgically placed gastrostomy or jejunostomy tube for nutritional support, since placement of an enteral feeding tube via the nasogastric route is not practical. The development of an endoscopic technique for the placement of a gastrostomy tube has been a very useful adjunct in the management of such patients and is rapidly becoming the treatment of choice. In this chapter, the two major techniques of percutaneous endoscopic gastrostomy (PEG) are outlined.

Indications

1. To provide an access for nutritional support in patients with an abnormality of the swallowing mechanism or in whom oral intake of food is precluded and long-term placement of an enteral feeding tube is not satisfactory.
2. Patients who demonstrate a potential for response to nutritional support.

Contraindications

1. Ascites.
2. Morbid obesity.
3. Extensive scarring of the anterior abdominal wall.

4. Significant bleeding diathesis.
5. Gastric outlet obstruction.

Preparation

1. Obtain surgical back-up.
2. Obtain operative consent by the patient or if necessary by a responsible family member.
3. Nothing by mouth (NPO) for 12 hr.
4. Place an i.v. to administer meperidine and midazolam or diazepam and atropine.
5. Remove dentures.
6. Administer prophylactic antibiotics, such as ampicillin or a cephalosporin.

Equipment

1. Upper endoscope and teaching attachment or video.
2. Topical anesthetic, tongue blades, and emesis basin.
3. Polyp snare and alligator grasping forceps.
4. Bite block and lubricant.
5. Gastrostomy-related equipment:

   a. Disposable lap pack;
   b. prep tray, including razor, alcohol, Betadine and sterile sponge sticks;
   c. suture tray with a No. 11 scalpel;
   d. masks, caps, boots, and sterile gloves;
   e. 1% Xylocaine with syringe and 25-gauge needle;
   f. 2-0 silk on a curved needle that is used to sew the bolster to the abdominal wall;
   g. No. 2 Dermalon to thread through the medicut;
   h. No. 14 and No. 16 medicut tapered i.v. catheters;
   i. No. 16 Malecot or mushroom Silastic catheter with the flared connection end cut off;
   j. a flared Christmas tree adapter for the cut end of the Silastic catheter;
   k. two 2-in.-long pieces of rubber tubing with short lengthwise slits to serve as bolsters to be placed over the Malecot Silastic catheter.

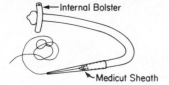

FIG. 1. Malecot catheter adapted for use with medicut sheath and internal bolster in place.

The Malecot catheter is prepared for use as the gastrostomy tube by cutting off the flared end and passing a Dermalon suture through the wall of the catheter near the cut end (but not so near that firm pulling might tear the catheter). Remove the needle from the suture material and pull the ends of the suture to equal lengths and tie a secure knot. Pass a medicut sheath over this suture so that it fits snugly over the cut end of the Malecot catheter. Slide one of the rubber bolsters with a small central slit over the Malecot catheter down to the mushroom end; this will then serve as the internal bolster (Fig. 1).

Procedure

1. Place the patient in approximately a 10° to 15° head-up, supine recumbent position. With the patient in this position, the team must carefully observe for the possibility of aspiration. Frequent suction may be needed.
2. If the patient is not cooperative, arm restraint with a blanket may be needed.
3. Prep the abdomen first using alcohol and then Betadine in circular motions, beginning from the proposed gastrostomy site and working outward. Drape the abdomen with towel drapes and a lap sheet.
4. Perform a standard diagnostic upper endoscopy (see Chapter 12) and identify the site for the gastrostomy tube. This site is located approximately one-third the distance from the left costal margin to the umbilicus. It is chosen by inflating the stomach in a darkened room, transilluminating the abdominal wall in the appropriate chosen area and then having the assistant push in the anterior abdominal wall so that one can see the finger indenting the anterior wall of the stomach.

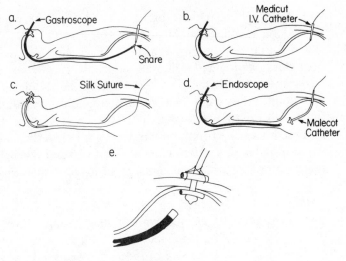

FIG. 2.

5. Pass the snare through the biopsy channel of the scope and position it near the chosen gastrostomy site.

6. Inject several cubic centimeters of Xylocaine into the anterior abdominal wall and make a skin incision. Thrust the medicut catheter in a perpendicular direction through the stab wound and through the anterior wall of the stomach. Loop the medicut catheter with the snare.

7. Remove the needle stylet of the catheter and pass a 60-in. silk suture through the catheter into the stomach.

8. At this point, the suture is grasped in the polyp snare. Tighten the snare around the silk suture (Fig. 2a).

9. Retract the endoscope, snare, and suture in tandem and pull them through the patient's mouth (Fig. 2b).

10. Remove the medicut catheter from the stomach. At this time, the silk suture can be seen exiting the anterior abdominal wall with the other end emerging from the patient's mouth.

11. Tie the previously prepared Malecot catheter to the suture exiting the patient's mouth.

12. With the Malecot catheter well lubricated, grasp the silk suture exiting the anterior abdominal wall and pull firmly

so the gastrostomy tube progresses sequentially through the mouth, esophagus, and stomach (Fig. 2c).

13. When the tapered tip of the medicut sheath begins to exit the anterior abdominal wall, reintroduce the endoscope to observe the gastrostomy catheter exiting the esophagus and monitor the positioning of the internal bolster against the anterior gastric wall (Fig. 2d).

14. Pull the bolster up firmly but not too tightly. If resistance is felt in pulling the knot or the Malecot catheter through the anterior abdominal wall, enlarge the skin incision (Fig. 2e).

15. Remove the endoscope.

16. Slide the external bolster down over the exiting gastrostomy tube and suture it in place with 2-0 silk.

17. Place an adapter at the end of the gastrostomy tube and attach it to straight drainage.

Procedure 2: Prepackaged System

With this system, the gastrostomy tube is placed using a modified peel-away sheath over a guide wire. A Foley catheter is then inserted directly through the peel-away sheath. [Prepackaged kits are available from Cook Critical Care, P.O. Box 489, Bloomington, Indiana 47402, (812) 339-2235.]

1. After endoscopically selecting and anesthetizing the gastrostomy site, advance an 18-gauge needle through the site into the stomach.

2. Insert a flexible J guide wire through the needle into the stomach and remove the needle.

3. Make a small incision adjacent to the guide wire with a blade 11 scalpel. This incision should be large enough to allow easy passage of the dilator and sheath.

4. Lubricate the lumen of the modified 16-French peel-away sheath, and with the dilator acting as an obturator pass the unit over the guide wire (Fig. 3a).

5. Under endoscopic observation, advance as a unit the wire guide, the dilator, and the peel-away sheath into the stomach. Use a rotary motion to facilitate passage.

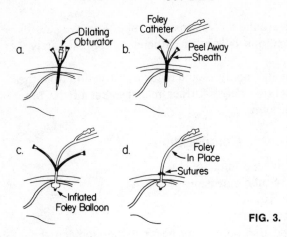

FIG. 3.

6. Remove the wire guide and dilator, leaving only the peel-away sheath in the stomach.
7. Lubricate a 14-French Foley catheter and advance it through the sheath until it is seen in the stomach (Fig. 3b).
8. Inflate the Foley balloon with 5 cc water to check the competency of the valve as well as the integrity of the balloon.
9. After confirming that the system is leakproof, peel the sheath away and remove it (Fig. 3c).
10. Bring the Foley catheter into aposition with the anterior abdominal wall by applying slight tension.
11. Suture the catheter to the anterior abdominal wall (Fig. 3d).

Postprocedure

1. Place the gastrostomy tube on straight drainage.
2. Give nothing by mouth except for medications for the next 24 hr. After this period, feeding via the gastrostomy tube may begin, provided that bowel sounds are normal and the patient is afebrile.
3. Flush the gastrostomy tube with 50 cc of tap water every 4 hr.
4. Change the gastrostomy site dressings daily for 3 days and then remove. This is accomplished by cleansing the wound with hydrogen peroxide and normal saline and then placing

slit 4 × 4's around the gastrostomy tube. Remove sutures from the external bolster or catheter in approximately 7 days.

5. The patient and family should receive instruction from the nutrition service about further management of the tube feedings at home.

Complications

1. Superficial wound infections.
2. Gastrostomy tube extrusions.
3. Gastrocolic fistula.
4. Pneumoperitoneum.
5. Leakage and peritonitis may occur if the stomach separates from the peritoneum and anterior abdominal wall.
6. Aspiration during the procedure.

REFERENCES

1. Ponsky JL, Gauderer MWL, Stellata TA (1983): Percutaneous endoscopic gastrostomy. *Arch Surg* 118:913–914.
2. Strodel WE, Lemmer J, Eckhauser F, Botham M, Dent T (1983): Early experience with endoscopic percutaneous gastrostomy. *Arch Surg* 118:449–453.
3. Ponsky JL (1984): Percutaneous endoscopic gastrostomy and jejunostomy: endoscopic highlights. *Gastrointest Endosc* 30:306–307.
4. Russell TR, Brotman M, Norris F (1984): Percutaneous gastrostomy. A new simplified and cost-effective technique. *Am J Surg* 148:132–137.
5. Stassen WN, McCullough AJ, Marshall JB, Eckhauser ML (1984): Percutaneous endoscopic gastrostomy: another cause of "benign" pneumoperitoneum. *Gastrointest Endosc* 30:296–298.
6. Ponsky JL (1985): Endoscopic placement of intestinal tubes. In: *Therapeutic Gastrointestinal Endoscopy*, edited by S.E. Silvis, pp. 94–113. Igaku-Shoin, New York.

31 / Endoscopic Sphincterotomy

Eugene M. Bozymski and Douglas A. Drossman

Endoscopic sphincterotomy is extremely useful in a number of clinical settings. The procedure has virtually replaced surgery for removal of common duct stones in the patient who has previously undergone cholecystectomy. Endoscopic sphincterotomy may also be useful for removal of common duct stones in the patient with an intact gallbladder at high surgical risk. For, when the symptom complex relates primarily to the common duct stones rather than to gallbladder disease, sphincterotomy may be all that is necessary. Another common indication for sphincterotomy is in the preparation for placement of a large stent to relieve neoplastic obstruction of the bile duct.

Dissolution therapy, primarily with monooctanoin and lithotripsy via extracorporeal and endoscopic techniques are other modalities for managing common duct stones. Their benefits relative to surgery or sphincterotomy will depend on the results of future clinical trials.

The solution to the problem of how best to teach and learn endoscopic sphincterotomy has not been adequately addressed. Endoscopic sphincterotomy should not be done by the physician until the skills of selective cannulation of the common bile duct have been mastered. Most often, this level of skill cannot be developed during the usual fellowship period. This training may best be accomplished by having selected fellows stay an additional year in therapeutic endoscopy or by having gastroenterologists return to the training center for further training in endoscopic sphincterotomy after acquiring more experience with ERCP.

Indications

1. Gallstones in the common bile duct.
   a. When the gallbladder has previously been removed.
   b. When the gallbladder is present: (i) in the patient at high surgical risk; (ii) may be indicated in the patient with acute illness (pancreatitis, cholangitis) prior to surgery.
2. To treat distal common bile duct obstruction: (a) surgical stricture; (b) well-documented ampullary stenosis; (c) ampullary tumor; and choledochocele.
3. Preliminary to the placement of common bile duct stents.
4. Preliminary to choledochoscopy.

Contraindications

Absolute

1. Impossible access to the papilla.
2. Inadequate training, equipment, or support personnel.

Relative

1. Coagulopathy.
2. Large stone size (>15 mm).
3. Long stricture.
4. Marked portal hypertension.

Preparation

1. Examine the patient and review the clinical data and laboratory studies to be certain that endoscopic sphincterotomy is the treatment of choice.
2. Obtain surgical back-up.
3. Send a blood clot to the blood bank for typing and cross-match testing if necessary.
4. Make certain that there is no contrast material in the gastrointestinal tract to obscure the area under evaluation.
5. Obtain informed, written consent.
6. Apply the grounding plate on the patient and check that the circuit in the sphincterotome is functioning properly.

7. Place an i.v. in the right arm with the fork close to the vein for administering atropine, meperidine, diazepam, or midazolam and glucagon.
8. Place the patient on preprocedure systemic antibiotics (aminoglycoside with or without a cephalosporin) if cholangitis or obstruction of the biliary tree or infection in the pancreas is suspected.
9. Have the patient lie on the left side with the left arm behind the back to facilitate the roll to the prone position after insertion of the duodenoscope into the duodenum.

Equipment

1. Duodenoscope.
2. Teaching attachment or video system.
3. A variety of cannulas (1.7 mm × 200 cm) with both blunt and tapered tips.
4. Renograffin at concentrations of 60% and 30%.
5. Several different papillotomes are available:

   a. Traction type (Demling-Classen):

   regular—wire ends 3–4 mm from tip;
   precut—wire ends at tip of papillotome;
   long nose—wire reenters cannula 3 cm from tip.

   b. Push type (Soma).
   c. Billroth II type—reverse-wire placement.
   d. Needle knife.

6. Balloon catheter and Dormia basket for removing stones.
7. Electrosurgical generating unit.
8. Patient grounding plate.
9. A fluoroscope with good image intensification on a TV monitoring system with capability for taking spot films.
10. X-ray cassettes.
11. Lead aprons and thyroid shields.
12. Gloves, lubricant, syringes, and needles.

Procedure

The physician performing the sphincterotomy should be versed in the anatomy of the biliary tree and have extensive endoscopic experience and skill in the use of electrocautery techniques. A guiding principle behind sphincterotomy is that the length of the incision be based on the reasons for the procedure. For example, the incision length should be long enough (usually 12–13 cm) to allow passage of the largest stone in the common duct as judged by the cholangiogram (with size corrected for magnification) but not so long that it extends beyond the intraduodenal portion of the common duct. When removing small stones, or when placing stents or treating ampullary stenosis, the excision length may be somewhat smaller. The physician should remain familiar with the power output settings on the electrosurgical generating unit. In our unit the power settings are similar to those we use for polypectomy.

1. Proceed with ERCP to obtain a cholangiogram and, if needed, a pancreatogram. Determine the anatomy of the ampulla of Vater and the puncta and the direction required for insertion of the cannula into the common bile duct. This will greatly assist in guiding the sphincterotome into the common duct.

2. Exchange the cannula for a sphincterotome and pass it into the duodenum. While working in the "short-stick" position (see Chapter 14), make certain that the ampulla is close up and properly aligned. Recall the direction of the common bile duct and with the sphincterotome thus directed, insert it for a short distance into the puncta. Inject some dye to make certain that the sphincterotome is in the common bile duct. Continue to insert the sphincterotome well into the common bile duct.

3. Have the assistant open the sphincterotome (making certain that the wire comes out in the 10 to 2 o'clock position relative to the ampulla of Vater). No more than 1.5 cm of wire should be in contact with the intraduodenal segment of the common bile duct. The wire should not be too taut. Rather, gently lift the ampulla of vater into the lumen of the duodenum. This allows for close contact of the wire with all parts of the ampulla and permits a more controlled cut to be made in the longitudinal axis of the intraduodenal portion of the common bile duct.

4. Begin the incision with no more than 1.5 cm of the wire within the ampulla. Bow the wire in the properly flexed position with respect to its tension on the ampulla by manipulating the tip of the scope as well as by changing the up–down lever of the sphincterotome. The exposed wire should not be in contact with the tip of the scope, as this will cause current leakage.

5. If the sphincterotome comes out of the common bile duct, reinsert and check fluoroscopically for placement prior to any actual cutting.

6. Apply short bursts (1–3 sec) of coagulation current while maintaining upward pressure on the wire until white coagulated tissue is seen near the wire. If there is a great deal of fluid present, more heat will be required. Following this, apply short bursts of blended cut current to lengthen the incision in 2- to 3-mm increments until the planned length of incision is achieved. Some physicians use only the blended cut current to make their sphincterotomy incisions; however, small quantities of coagulation current minimize the chance of bleeding. Too much coagulation current will increase tissue resistance and prevent a controlled incision.

7. Occasionally, when flexing the sphincterotome within the ampulla of Vater, it will back out into the duodenal lumen. Halt this process by having the assistant decrease the flex of the sphincterotome wire and then reinsert the wire. If the incision is being made too rapidly, the assistant should decrease the flexion on the sphincterotome. If bleeding occurs, follow with a little coagulation current along the edges of the cut. Most bleeding is clinically insignificant. With rapid bleeding, the endoscopist may try tamponading with a balloon catheter or injecting 1/10,000 epinephrine into the bleeding area.

8. If on occasion the sphincterotome will not advance into the common bile duct, several maneuvers may be tried:

   a. make to and fro lateral movements of the sphincterotome within the common duct while exerting gentle forward pressure with the right hand;

b. make up and down movements with the left thumb on the endoscope elevator while advancing the sphincterotome;

c. reposition the scope tip to recannulate from a different orientation relative to the papilla;

d. on rare occasions, make a small precut to introduce the sphincterotome into the common bile duct (this procedure is associated with a higher complication rate and should not be done until the physician is experienced in sphincterotomy);

e. at times the sphincterotome can be advanced fluoroscopically by moving the tip of the sphincterotome into a more favorable position within the lumen of the common duct rather than along its wall. Insert the sphincterotome only for very short distances before fluoroscopically checking sphincterotome position to avoid placing the sphincterotome into the pancreatic duct.

9. Compare the size of the stones (corrected for magnification) as seen on the cholangiogram with the length of the sphincterotomy using the size of the duodenoscope as a reference measurement. If the sphincterotomy length is considered large enough to permit stone passage, insert a balloon catheter into the common bile duct above the stone; inflate it and pull it down into the duodenal lumen with the stone before it. When the common bile duct is greatly dilated, the stones may slide alongside the balloon into the more proximal common bile duct. When this occurs, try to capture the stones with a biliary basket (Fig. 1). Again, be certain that the sphincterotomy size is larger than the entrapped stone. If basket retrieval is to be attempted, we recommend that stone-crushing baskets be available. If the balloon readily passes through the sphincterotomy and is larger than the largest stone, terminate the procedure and await spontaneous passage of the stones. The stool can be strained over the ensuing days to retrieve the stones.

10. If any stones remain at the end of the procedure, place a nasobiliary tube (see Chapter 32) for decompression and reevaluate in several days.

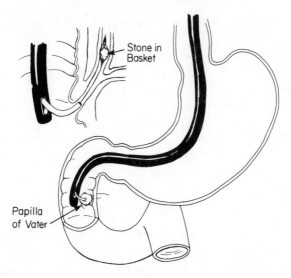

FIG. 1. Papillotomy.

11. Because of the reverse direction of approach, sphincterotomy is particularly difficult (but not impossible) in the patient with a Billroth II gastrectomy and is associated with a higher complication rate. While forward-viewing endoscopes have been recommended to permit better visualization, cannulation is problematic, since there is no elevator. Recently, the use of the wide-angle side-viewing endoscopes with retrograde lens systems and Billroth II reverse-wire papillotomes have considerably increased the success rate. Sphincterotomy is also more difficult if the patient has undergone previous surgery in the duodenal area such as a choledochoduodenostomy or if there is anatomic distortion by tumor and may be more difficult if periampullary diverticula are present.

Postprocedure

1. Monitor vital signs.
2. Clear liquid diet for the remainder of the day and then resume regular diet.

3. Bathroom privileges for 6 hr postprocedure; then ambulation ad lib.
4. Maintain an i.v. with D5W.
5. Serum amylase in 6 hr and again the following morning.
6. Hematocrit the following morning.
7. If done for common bile duct stones, strain all stool for stones.
8. If there has been extensive manipulation of the common bile duct and residual stones are present, broad-spectrum antibiotics are continued.

Complications

The complication rate ranges up to 11% with a 30-day mortality of 1.4%. These rates vary directly with the age of the patient and inversely with the experience of the endoscopist.

Immediate

1. Bleeding (up to 5%). Most severe episodes occur immediately.
2. Perforation (up to 2%). Due to improper cut angle, long incision, small common bile duct, or forceful stone-pulling.
3. Stone impaction.
4. Oversedation.

Delayed

1. Cholangitis (up to 5%). Requires repeat effort to remove the stones or achieve tube drainage.
2. Pancreatitis (up to 3%).
3. Bleeding.
4. Cholecystitis (if gallbladder present).
5. Impaction of stone in distal duct or distal ileum.

REFERENCES

1. Zimmon DS (1984): Devices and techniques for endoscopic sphincterotomy (editorial). *Gastrointest Endosc* 30:214–215.
2 Siegel JH (1983): Instrumentation evaluation: endoscopic retro-

grade cholangiopancreatography and endoscopic sphincterotomy. *Gastrointest Endosc* 29:42–44.

3. Vennes JA (1983): Management of calculi in the common duct. *Semin Liver Dis* 3:162–171.

4. Silvis SE, Vennes JA (1985): Endoscopic retrograde sphincterotomy. In: *Therapeutic Gastrointestinal Endoscopy*, edited by SE Silvis, pp. 198–240. Igaku-Shoin, New York.

5. Geenen JE (1982): New diagnostic and treatment modalities involving endoscopic retrograde cholangiopancreatography and esophagogastroduodenoscopy. *Scan J Gastroenterol Suppl* 77:93.

6. Siegel JH (1980): Endoscopy and papillotomy in diseases of the biliary tract and pancreas. *J. Clin Gastroenterol* 2:337.

7. Cotton PB (1980): Nonoperative removal of bile duct stones by duodenoscopic sphincterotomy. *Br J Surg* 67:1.

8. Safrany L, Cotton PB (1982): Endoscopic management of choledocholithiasis. *Surg Clin North Am* 62:825.

32 / Endoscopic Biliary Decompression: Nasobiliary Tube

Eugene M. Bozymski

Although there are now many ways to achieve decompression of an obstructed biliary tree, the advantages of using the nasobiliary tube are (a) it is relatively simple to insert, and (b) once in place, cholangiograms may be obtained at any time to check the status of the biliary system. Additionally, the nasobiliary tube may be used to perfuse monooctanoin in selected cases in which common bile duct stones are refractory to removal.

Indications

Nasobiliary drains are used for temporary decompression of an obstructed or partially obstructed common bile duct. Examples include (a) retained stones present after endoscopic sphincterotomy; and (b) decompression of a biliary stricture (e.g., pancreatic mass) prior to surgery.

Contraindications

There are no absolute contraindications, except for technical inaccessibility of the ampulla of Vater.

Preparation

1. Perform an endoscopic retrograde cholangeopancreatogram (ERCP) (see Chapter 14).

2. Administer broad-spectrum antibiotics in the periprocedure period. An aminoglycoside and a cephalosporin (or a third-generation cephalosporin with pseudomonas coverage) are appropriate.

Equipment

1. Same equipment as that used for an ERCP (see Chapter 14).
2. Select any of several nasobiliary catheters (5–7 French, 250–300 cm) and guidewires as clinically indicated.
3. Silicone lubricant.
4. A small Foley catheter or nasogastric tube for changing the orobiliary catheter into a nasobiliary catheter.

Procedure

1. Initially, we modify our standard blunt-tipped ERCP cannula by enlarging its opening to approximately an 18-gauge needle size. Alternatively, a slightly larger ERCP cannula may be used.
2. Cannulate the common bile duct and using fluoroscopic guidance, slide the catheter as high into the biliary tree as possible.
3. Insert a guidewire of at least 300 cm in length through the ERCP cannula into the common bile duct and intrahepatic radicles. This is facilitated by initially placing a drop of silicone lubricant over the guidewire.
4. Carefully remove the ERCP catheter while maintaining the guidewire deep within a biliary radical. Gradually retract the catheter as an assistant simultaneously feeds the guidewire into the channel. Monitor fluoroscopically to maintain position of the guidewire.
5. If the guidewire does not slide through the standard (1.7-mm sheath) ERCP cannula, place a Soehendra dilating biliary catheter into the common bile duct and insert the guidewire through this and then remove the Soehendra dilating catheter.
6. Insert the nasobiliary catheter over the guidewire. It is helpful if the guidewire and catheter are of different colors.

Keep the guidewire tight and lubricate it with silicone lubricant.

7. Keep the tip of the endoscope very close to the ampulla of Vater so that forward pressure will be directed upward into the common bile duct rather than downward into the duodenum, thus forming a loop within the duodenum. Monitor the advancement of the tube via fluoroscopy.

8. Manipulate the elevator repeatedly in the upward direction to maintain the progress of the nasobiliary catheter as it proceeds to the proximal bile duct.

9. Using fluoroscopic guidance, pull back the guidewire into the nasobiliary catheter to a point several centimeters below the pigtail portion and gradually remove the scope while simultaneously advancing the nasobiliary catheter through the channel at the same rate. With one-to-one movement, the position of the nasobiliary catheter within the common bile duct will not change.

10. Do not remove the endoscope and guidewire until the nasobiliary catheter is in place in the proximal portion of the biliary tree.

11. Once the endoscope is removed, adjust the nasobiliary catheter to its proper position in the biliary tree and along the duodenal and gastric walls and then remove the guidewire using silicone lubricant.

12. The nasobiliary tube now exits from the mouth and must be transferred to exit from the nose for greater patient acceptance. Pass a small soft Foley catheter or nasogastric tube through the nose, pick its end up in the pharynx and pull it out through the mouth. Cut off the excess portion of the nasobiliary tube. Thread the nasobiliary tube up through the Foley catheter that exits out of the mouth into the proximal portion of the catheter that exits through the nose. Reduce the slack of the nasobiliary cannula by pulling on it as it emerges through the Foley catheter. Fluoroscopically check the position of the distal end of the nasobiliary catheter (Fig. 1).

13. Attach a leuerlock to the nasobiliary catheter and connect to a Foley bag for straight drainage.

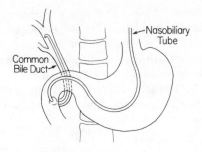

FIG. 1. Position of the nasobiliary drain through the stomach and duodendum into the common bile duct.

Postprocedure

1. Monitor as for ERCP (see Chapter 14).
2. Attach the nasobiliary catheter to straight drainage and using sterile technique, flush once or twice daily.
3. The nasobiliary catheter may be used for repeat cholangiograms as necessary.

Complications

Complications generally relate to the performance of the ERCP (see Chapter 14).

REFERENCES

1. Vennes JA (1983): Management of calculi in the common duct. *Semin Liver Dis* 3:162–171.
2. Venu RP, Geenen JE, Toouli J, Hogan WJ, Kozlov N, Stewart ET (1982): Gallstone dissolution using mono-octanoin infusion through an endoscopically placed nasobiliary catheter. *Am J Gastroenterol* 77:227–230.
3. Leuschner U, Wurbs D, Baumgartel H, Helm EB, Classen M (1981): Alternating treatment of common bile duct stones with a modified glyceryl-1-monooctanoate preparation and bile acid-EDTA solution by nasobiliary tube. *Scand J Gastroenterol* 16:497–503.
4. Demling L (1983): Therapeutic endoscopy. *Acta Med Austriaca* 10:93–99.

5. Wurbs D, Phillip J, Classen M (1980): Experiences with longstanding nasobiliary tube in biliary disease. *Endoscopy* 12:219–223.
6. Siegel JH (1985): Endoscopic decompression of the biliary tree. In: *Therapeutic Gastrointestinal Endoscopy,* edited by SE Silvis, pp. 241–268. Igaku-Shoin, New York and Tokyo.
7. Soehendra N, Reynders-Frederix V (1980): Palliative bile duct drainage: a new endoscopic method of introducing a transpapillary drain. *Endoscopy* 12:8–11.

33 / Endoscopic Biliary Decompression: Endoprostheses

Eugene M. Bozymski and Douglas A. Drossman

The ability to place endoprostheses or stents endoscopically into the biliary tree has had considerable impact on the management of obstructing bile duct lesions. During the past several years, this procedure has become the preferred treatment for palliation of obstructing malignant pancreatic or biliary tumors. Endoprostheses are available in a variety of shapes, lengths, and diameters. They range from single- and double-pigtail types to straight stents with side flaps (Amsterdam) (Fig. 1). Endoprostheses up to 7 French can be placed through the standard duodenoscope (2.8-mm channel), whereas the larger duodenoscope (4.2-mm channel) is necessary for placement of the 10 and 11.5 French endoprostheses. The smaller prostheses are easier to place but become clogged relatively quickly, and recent data suggest that the rate of cholangitis is higher. The larger prostheses are therefore generally preferred; however, they require a sphincterotomy and the use of a coaxial system with an intermediate-size catheter threaded between the guide wire and stent/pusher system.

Indications

1. To alleviate obstructive jaundice secondary to unresectable pancreatic cancer in which there is no gastric outlet obstruction.
2. To alleviate obstruction due to biliary neoplasms not amenable to surgical correction (e.g., hilar tumors).
3. To alleviate biliary obstruction due to certain benign strictures (e.g., chronic pancreatitis, sclerosing cholangitis).

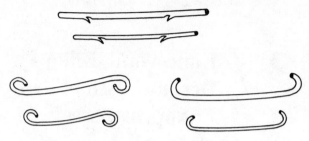

FIG. 1. A variety of endoprotheses.

4. To provide biliary decompression and prevent impaction after sphincterotomy and attempted extraction when gallstones remain in the common bile duct.

Contraindications

1. See also Chapter 31, Endoscopic Sphincterotomy.
2. Obstruction due to multiple intrahepatic strictures.

Preparation

1. Generally, the same preparation as is necessary for endoscopic retrograde cholangiopancreatography (ERCP) and sphincterotomy (see Chapters 14 and 31).
2. Broad-spectrum antibiotic coverage (e.g., aminoglycoside and a cephalosporin or a third-generation cephalosporin with pseudomonas coverage is usually indicated).
3. It is essential that the surgical and radiological consultants be involved in deciding on the course of treatment. We also recommend that the radiologist be in attendance during the procedure.

Equipment

The equipment is the same as that required for ERCP and endoscopic sphincterotomy (see Chapters 14 and 31). In addition, the following should also be available:

1. A wide selection of endoprostheses of varying diameters (7, 10, and 11.5 French) and lengths (5–15 cm measured

between the flanges) may be used. These are available in sets with accompanying guide wire (400 cm or greater recommended) and pusher cannulas of various colors.

2. Dilating biliary catheters (e.g., Soehendra type) of varying diameters (5–12 French).

Procedure

Successful endoprosthesis placement requires close coordination among the physician and at least two assistants during the procedure: one assists with the equipment and the other monitors the patient.

1. Perform a diagnostic ERCP (see Chapter 14).
2. After obtaining the cholangiogram, choose the appropriate-length endoprosthesis, depending on the evident pathology and anatomic configuration of the common bile duct. We use the straight endoprosthesis with side flaps (Amsterdam) most often. The method of inserting an endoprosthesis is similar to that used for inserting a nasobiliary drain (see Chapter 32).
3. Perform a sphincterotomy (see Chapter 31) if a large endoprosthesis is to be used or if the anatomical situation requires one prior to the placement of the endoprosthesis.
4. Advance the guide wire (0.035 in. × 400 cm) well into the intrahepatic bile radicals.
5. If traversing the narrowed area appears difficult, thread the Soehendra biliary dilating catheters over the guide wire and across the lesion until the segment is dilated to the size of the endoprosthesis to be used.
6. Based on anatomy and clinical need, choose the appropriate endoprosthesis. For the smaller (7 French) endoprosthesis, mount the tapered end directly onto the guide wire and advance it into the endoscope using a pushing catheter of the same size but of a different color than the endoprosthesis. With the 10 and 11.5 French coaxial system, thread a 6.5 French inner catheter over the guide wire and advance it through the stricture. Dilators can then be threaded over the catheter as needed. Following this, at-

tach the prostheses (tapered end first) and pusher and advance it over the catheter and into the endoscope.

7. Once the endoprosthesis is in the shaft of the endoscope it cannot be retracted. Therefore, it is important to have the tip of the scope very close to the ampulla of Vater so that when the endoprosthesis comes into view it is close enough to the puncta to be directed cephalad without pulling the guide wire back into the duodenum.

8. As the prosthesis emerges from the scope (recognized by its different color), continue to advance it into the common bile duct as the assistant pulls back on the guide wire (or guide-wire/inner catheter system). Use the elevator frequently to keep proper angulation of the prosthesis relative to the common bile duct. Silicone lubricant should be used to decrease friction between the guide wire and the pusher cannula. If the direction of force of the pusher tube exerted on the endoprosthesis is incorrect, the guide wire will form a loop in the duodenum and will begin to back out of the common bile duct. This problem can be minimized by monitoring the procedure fluoroscopically and by having the assistant keep the guide wire taut. If looping occurs, have the assistant gently pull back on the guide wire to reduce the slack. Fluoroscopically monitor the distal end for any slippage that might occur.

9. When the prosthesis is securely in place, have the assistant remove the guide wire (and catheter) as you hold the prosthesis in place by using forward pressure on the pusher. As the guide wire exits the duodenal end of the endoprosthesis, the pusher rod and the endoprosthesis are separated. Final adjustment of the tip of the endoprosthesis can be made by using the pusher cannula that is seen at the tip of the endoscope.

10. Observe the patient for bile flow and fluoroscopically recheck the placement of the stent before removing the endoscope.

11. Depending on the clinical situation, we recommend that the stent be replaced between 4 and 6 months to prevent later complications, such as clogging or fracture.

Postprocedure

1. Monitor the patient's status as per sphincterotomy and nasobiliary stent placement (see Chapters 31 and 32).
2. Obtain serial liver chemistries to monitor the adequacy of the biliary decompression.
3. The patency of the endoprosthesis may later be determined with radionuclide scanning. Alternatively, another ERCP can be done by inserting a cannula into the tip of the endoprosthesis and injecting contrast. It is not known whether or not placing the patient on long-term cheno- or ursodeoxycholic acid is of added benefit in maintaining patency of the endoprosthesis.

Complications

The complication rate ranges from 5% to 30%, depending on the skill of the physician, the size of the endoprosthesis (fewer complications with larger stents), and the location (fewer complications with distal lesions) and number of obstructing lesions.

Early Complications

1. Cholangitis.
2. Dislocation.
3. Hemobilia.
4. Perforation.

Late Complications

1. Clogging of tube.
2. Cholangitis.
3. Liver or pancreatic abscess.
4. Fracture.
5. Cholecystitis.
6. Perforation.

BIBLIOGRAPHY

Laurence BH, Cotton PB (1980): Decompression of malignant biliary obstruction by duodenoscopic intubation of bile ducts. *Br Med J* 280:522–523.

Huibregtse K, Tytgat GN: Palliative treatment of obstructive jaundice by transpapillary introduction of large bore bile duct endoprosthesis. *Gut* 23:371–375.

Siegel JH, Harding GT, Chateau F (1982): Endoscopic decompression and drainage of benign and malignant biliary obstruction. *Gastrointest Endosc* 28:79–82.

Siegel JH, Yatto RP (1983): Approach to cholestasis: an update. *Arch Intern Med* 142:1877–1879.

Siegel JH (1985): Endoscopic decompression of the biliary tree. In: *Therapeutic Gastrointestinal Endoscopy,* edited by SE Silvis, pp. 241–268. Igaku-Shoin, New York and Tokyo.

34 / Colonoscopic Polypectomy

Douglas A. Drossman

Colonoscopic polypectomy is a procedure that is diagnostic; therapeutic; cost-effective, when compared to surgery; and very likely prophylactic for colon cancer (1). [*Note.* All information in Chapter 15, Colonoscopy, applies here. More detailed discussion of polypectomy technique can be found elsewhere (2,3).]

Indication

Removal of colonic polyps not believed to be invasive polypoid carcinomas.

Contraindications

1. Evidence of a bleeding or coagulation disorder (see Chapter 22).
2. No available surgical backup for large polyps.
3. Poor bowel preparation.

Equipment

1. Coagulator and grounding plate.
2. Colon polyp snare, handle, and sheath.
3. Retrieval instrument (optional).

Preparation

There is a trend for colonoscopic polypectomy to be performed on an outpatient basis; however, we would recommend overnight hospitalization if the polyp or stalk is large or if complications arise during the procedure.

1. Explain the reasons for the procedure, possible complications, and alternative therapy. Obtain written consent.
2. Test the coagulation equipment to be certain it is in working order.
3. Start an i.v. and administer Meperidine and Diazepam or Midazolam as needed.
4. Check the patient's prothrombin time, platelet count, and hematocrit. (For patients with no historical reason for a bleeding disorder, these tests may be obtained up to 1 week prior to the procedure.)
5. Give SBE prophylaxis if indicated (see Colonoscopy, Chapter 15).

Procedure

1. Perform a complete colonoscopy (see Chapter 15, Colonoscopy).
2. Attach the ground plate to the patient's thigh.
3. Set the power level based on the manufacturer's recommendations and prior experience with your electrosurgical unit. More power and coagulation time are needed
   a. for larger polyps;
   b. when there is greater tissue resistance (occurs with dessication during coagulation);
   c. a larger diameter snare wire is used;
   d. there is less traction on the stalk; and
   e. when pure coagulation, rather than blended (cutting and coagulation), current is used.

   For average-sized polyps (1–2 cm), we usually perform polypectomy with a coagulation setting of $2\frac{1}{2}$ to $3\frac{1}{2}$ using a 0.42-mm Olympus snare and the Valley Lab Model SSE2 coagulator. If the stalk is very thick or if the snare cannot be pulled through easily, we may alternate between coagulation and brief bursts of cutting current. Use of pure cut increases the risk of bleeding complications.
4. Identify the polyp and determine if it is pedunculated or sessile. If this cannot easily be determined, manipulate the polyp or reposition the patient to obtain optimal visual-

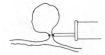

FIG. 1. Snare placement for polypectomy.

ization. Be certain there is no excess stool, mucus, or fluid present in the area.

5. Insert the snare catheter and advance through the colonoscope. Push out the wire to form a loop. Lasso the polyp and place the "V" of the snare on the stalk closer to the head of the polyp than the bowel wall. Ideally, the axis of the stalk should be the same as the snare, in the 6 o'clock position (Fig. 1).

6. Slowly tighten the snare around the stalk, being certain that the head of the polyp or bowel mucosa is not caught and that there is no contact of the polyp head with the opposite wall of the colon. The polyp head should start to turn a dusky blue.

7. Briefly coagulate ($\frac{1}{4}$–$\frac{1}{2}$ sec) and observe for a white area of burn on the stalk.

8. Coagulate while pulling the snare through. There should be a smooth but gradually resistive response. If a great deal of resistance is experienced, stop and reexamine for proper positioning of the snare and for blanching of the stalk. *Do not pull through without coagulation!*

9. If the polyp head unavoidably makes contact with the opposite wall, gently move the catheter back and forth during coagulation to maximize the area of burn contact.

10. In 2 or 3 sec the snare will "snap" when pulled through the stalk. Observe the stalk for bleeding or excess burn.

11. Remove the polyp by suction, snare, or retrieval instrument (Fig. 2).

12. If there is any question of a complication, reinsert the colonoscope and check the polypectomy site again.

13. If bleeding occurs and does not stop spontaneously, two techniques may be used:

    a. Resnare the stalk and tamponade for 5 to 10 min. Do not recoagulate with the snare.

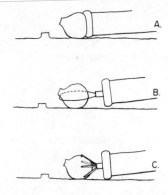

FIG. 2. Method for removal of transected polyps. Polyps may be suctioned (**A**), snared (**B**), or extracted by a pronged retrieval instrument (**C**).

b. Flush 1:10,000 dilution epinephrine through a catheter impacted into the stalk. This produces a "bleb" in the submucosa around the vessel and usually stops the bleeding.

On rare occasions, selective intraarterial perfusion of vasopressin, angiographic ablation of the feeding vessel, or surgical intervention is required.

Technique for Small Sessile Polyps (<1 cm)

Snare Cautery

The snare-cautery technique can be used to lasso the polyp at its base. Gentle tightening will produce a "pseudostalk" that can then be transected. The small arterial supply and the absence of a true stalk with these polyps makes the risk of transmural burn or perforation greater than bleeding. Therefore, we use a lower coagulation setting ($2\frac{1}{2}$). We routinely place a mucus trap in series with the suction tube to retrieve the polyp.

"Hot-Biopsy" Technique

The hot-biopsy technique can be used for lesions up to 8 mm. There is adequate, but incomplete sampling of tissue. When done effectively, the tissue not in the jaws of the forceps is coagulated. This method is quick and does not cause major bleeding difficulties:

1. Grasp the head of the polyp and pull away from the wall to make a "pseudostalk."
2. Coagulate ($2\frac{1}{2}$ setting) and observe for the white burn to extend into but not through the pseudostalk.
3. Do not attempt to burn off the polyp. With the jaws closed, pull off the sample and retrieve it.
4. Observe the area for bleeding or burn.

Technique for Large Sessile Polyps (>2 cm)

A clinical decision must be made with regard to the risks and benefits of polypectomy versus those of surgery. The procedure should not be performed if (a) the endoscopist is inexperienced; (b) the polyp appears to contain malignant tissue (ulcerated, friable, irregular contour); (c) the procedure will technically be difficult (poor visualization or ability to manipulate the snare effectively).

1. The polyp is removed in a piecemeal fashion by obliquely encircling one end of the base and placing the "V" of the wire near the top midportion of the polyp (Fig. 3a). No more than 30% of the polyp should be transected with each cut.
2. Coagulate and pull through the tissue.
3. Repeat the procedure at the other end of the polyp (Fig. 3b).
4. A pyramid of tissue will remain. Encircle at least the top half and coagulate it off (Fig. 3c,d).
5. Retrieve all pieces for histopathologic evaluation.
6. If the tissue is benign, colonoscopy should be repeated in 6 to 8 weeks to determine whether further resection is

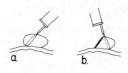
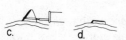

FIG. 3. Removal of large sessile polyp. **a:** Piecemeal removal of polyp. **b:** Procedure repeated at other end of polyp. **c,d:** Top half of polyp is encircled and coagulated off (see text).

needed. In many cases, the remaining tissue will have sloughed off. If the tissue is malignant, surgery is required.

Postprocedure

1. Fill out a procedure note indicating appearance, size, and location of polyp(s) removed.
2. Send polyp(s) to pathology in individually labeled formalin jars.
3. Check the patient's condition. Note particularly any areas of local abdominal pain or tenderness. Instruct the patient to report back if pain, bleeding, or fever occurs.

Complications (3)

Bleeding (1.7%)

Bleeding complications usually occur when inadequate coagulation is used for pedunculated polyps. It may be observed immediately, within the first 24 hr or in 5 to 7 days (when the fibrin clot falls off). Most bleeding episodes are self-limited and do not require further action.

Perforation (0.3%)

Perforation occurs most often when too much current is applied on sessile polyps or when a portion of adjacent colonic mucosa is transected. Exploratory laparotomy may need to be performed if perforation is clinically detected.

Transmural Burns ("Colon Coagulation Syndrome")

This occurs when the coagulation produces peritoneal inflammation without gross perforation. The patient has localized peritoneal signs, abdominal pain, fever, and leukocytosis within the first 24 hr. Surgery is usually not required. The patient should be made NPO. Observe for 1 to 2 days and administer i.v. fluids and antibiotics.

Explosion

Since colonic bacteria may produce combustible gases, explosion is a potential hazard. An adequate colonic prep with either cathartics/enemas or lavage solution is sufficient to eliminate this risk (4). We also recommend that carbohydrates be eliminated from the diets of patients about to have a polypectomy.

REFERENCES

1. Gilbertson VA, Nelms JM (1978): The prevention of invasive cancer of the rectum. *Cancer* 41:1137–1139.
2. Fruhmorgen P (1981): Therapeutic colonoscopy. In: *Colonscopy: Techniques, Clinical Practice and Colour Atlas*, edited by RH Hunt and JD Waye, pp 199–236. Chapman and Hall, London.
3. Tedesco FJ (1985): Colonoscopic polypectomy. In: *Therapeutic Gastrointestinal Endoscopy*, edited by SE Silvis, pp 269–288. Igaku-Shoin, New York.
4. DiPalma JA, Brady CE, Stewart DL, Karlin DA, et al. (1984): Comparison of colon cleansing methods in preparation for colonoscopy. *Gastroenterology* 86:856–860.

35 / Coagulation of Bleeding Gastrointestinal Lesions

Douglas A. Drossman

The methods commonly available for treating bleeding lesions of the gastrointestinal (GI) tract involve monopolar, bipolar, and thermal (e.g., Heat Probe) coagulation units.[1] The probes, which are attached to electrosurgical units, pass through the endoscope biopsy channel. All three techniques are effective in stopping bleeding from experimentally induced ulcers.

Monopolar Electrocoagulation

This involves generation of high-frequency electrical energy from the probe through the tissue to a distal electrode at a site on the patient's body. The depth of injury is difficult to regulate.

Bipolar Electrocoagulation

With this method, the potential for deep tissue injury is reduced, since the electrodes are limited to the area of the probe; however, a larger number of applications are usually needed to stop bleeding. The most popular bipolar electrode system is the BICAP (Microvasive, Milford, Massachusetts), which contains a circumferentially placed six-bipolar electrode oriented around a cylinder that is also attached to a water pump.

---

[1] Coagulation produces tissue necrosis without cutting either by fulguration (sparking of tissue) or dessication (no sparking—direct contact).

230

Direct Heat Thermal Cautery

Direct heat thermal cautery transfers energy to tissue by thermal conduction. The energy is diffused at a relatively low temperature (250°C), thereby limiting the potential for acute tissue erosion. We use the Heat Probe unit (Olympus Co., Lake Success, New York) almost exclusively for coagulation because

1. the depth of injury is limited to 1 to 3 mm;
2. there is little electrical hazard to the patient;
3. coagulation can occur with any angle of application;
4. the device is portable and inexpensive;
5. water flow and energy settings may be preset;
6. washing and tamponade can be done simultaneously; and
7. tissue adherance is minimized through use of the Teflon coating.

The probes come in 2.4- and 3.2-mm sizes.

Indications

1. To stop bleeding from gastrointestinal lesions:
    a. ulcers;
    b. arteriovenous malformations (angiodysplasia, telangiectasia);
    c. localized gastritis;
    d. Mallory-Weiss tears.
2. To prevent bleeding from lesions at high risk to bleed[2]:
    a. "visible vessels," sentinel clot, marginal oozing, "red spot" on an ulcer;
    b. arteriovenous malformations.

Contraindications

1. Unstable patient status.
2. Massively bleeding arterial lesions.

---

[2] In a retrospective evaluation of ten patients with nonbleeding visible vessels treated by heater probe, no patients rebled over 1 year, and an average of 4.1 U blood were required during hospitalization. Of eight patients with nonbleeding visible vessels *not treated* with heater probe, four patients rebled and went to surgery; this group averaged 10.8 U (5).

3. Bleeding from esophageal varices.
4. Arteriovenous malformations >1 cm may be difficult to ablate because of large submucosal feeding vessels.

Equipment

1. Large-channel endoscopes and accessory equipment (see Chapters 12 and 15).
2. Heat Probe and housing unit or monopolar or bipolar electrodes and transformer units.
3. Crash cart with cardiac monitoring unit.

Preparation

1. Pretest all electrical equipment to ensure that it is in proper working order. Attach the distant electrode for monopolar coagulation.
2. Be certain that the patient is clinically stable.
3. Remove blood and clots, using a large Edlich tube if there is gastroduodenal bleeding or, if possible, administer a Golytely prep for colonic bleeding.

Procedure

1. Perform an emergency upper endoscopy (see Chapter 12) or colonoscopy (see Chapter 15) to confirm the site of bleeding and to identify other gastrointestinal lesions.
2. Decide which lesions will be coagulated. In our unit, we coagulate actively bleeding lesions and usually coagulate certain high-risk nonbleeding lesions (visible vessel, "red spot" on ulcer, etc.).
3. Set the energy level based on manufacturer's recommendations and previous experience with the technique and coagulation unit (see Heat Probe Applications for Specific Lesions).
4. Wash away any blood or clot from the area to be coagulated. Do not apply energy pulses through blood, since this produces a coagulum that will raise tissue impedance. If blood is seen oozing from a clot in the base of an ulcer, gently dislodge and lift away the clot with the probe.

5. Coagulate the bleeding site. With the Heat Probe, apply firm pressure to the vessel sufficient to tamponade an actively bleeding lesion. Apply several heater probe pulses to coapt or seal the walls of the vessel. With the mono- or bipolar probes, first place the probe adjacent (~2 mm) to the vessel. Coagulate for 2 to 3 sec with each application and continue circumferentially. Finally, place the probe firmly on the vessel to finish. Initial direct electrocoagulation should only be attempted if the vessel is small (1–3 mm).

Heat Probe Applications for Specific Lesions

Bleeding Ulcer Vessels

For large arteries apply 20- to 30-Joule (J) pulses in three to six applications (up to 120 J). Circumferential application around larger vessels may also be done.

Angiodysplasia

For most lesions, apply 5- to 10-J pulses in one to three applications. Larger lesions (>7 mm in diameter) may first require circumferential applications beginning at the periphery.

Mallory-Weiss Tears

These lesions almost always require tangential application of the probe (60–90 J).

Complications

1. Continued or worsening of active bleeding.
2. Perforation.

BIBLIOGRAPHY

1. Swain CP, Mills TN, Shemesh E, et al. (1984): Which electrode? A comparison of four endoscopic methods of electrocoagulation in experimental bleeding ulcers. *Gut* 25:1424–1431.
2. Protell RL, Gilbert DA, Opie EA, et al. (1981): Computer-assisted

electrocoagulation: bipolar vs. monopolar in the treatment of experimental gastric ulcer bleeding. *Gastroenterology* 80:451–455.

3. Papp, JP (1985): Endoscopic management of gastrointestinal bleeding with electrocoagulation. In: *Therapeutic Gastrointestinal Endoscopy*, edited by SE Silvis, pp. 130–150. Igaku-Shoin, New York.

4. Sanowski RA (1986): Thermal application for gastrointestinal bleeding. *J Clin Gastroenterol* 8:239–244.

5. Jones S. (1986): Retrospective assessment of efficacy of heater probe treatment for nonbleeding "visible vessels": UNC experience. (*Personal communication.*)

36 / Unique Aspects of Gastrointestinal Procedures for Pediatric Patients

Martin H. Ulshen

Virtually any gastrointestinal (GI) procedure available for adults also can be performed in infants and children. Withholding a study only because of concern about the patient's size may, in fact, be detrimental to the child's care. On the other hand, some procedures are technically more difficult in children. In addition, even an experienced gastroenterologist may have difficulty if he or she is not comfortable working with children. For these reasons, there may be times when it is best to refer the patient to a physician with expertise in the field of pediatric gastroenterology.

Sedation

Procedures should be done under sedation only in an area where the proper equipment is available for resuscitation of the pediatric patient and where individuals familiar with pediatric resuscitation are readily available.

1. The greatest difficulty in working with infants and young children is their inability to comprehend and cooperate.
2. Children old enough to comprehend benefit from an explanation about the procedure in advance and often from a tour of the area where it will be done. Any facility where procedures are done regularly with children should have support from a play therapist. This therapist can help by reviewing the procedure with the child while he or she acts the part of the physician, using a doll as the patient.

3. Older children may need only this kind of introduction to tolerate the less uncomfortable tests, such as small bowel biopsy and sigmoidoscopy. One may also give an older child the choice as to whether he or she would prefer sedation.
4. The physician must be prepared to spend a greater amount of time performing a procedure in a child than might be necessary in an adult. It is best to explain each step of the procedure immediately before performance and to avoid sudden, unexpected movements.
5. Young children (i.e., <5 years of age) often need sedation or, rarely, general anesthesia, depending on the procedure.
6. For the procedures associated with the least discomfort, such as small bowel biopsy, sigmoidoscopy, or liver biopsy, milder sedation given 45 min or 1 hr before the procedure may be all that is necessary. *The dosage given below is for otherwise healthy children receiving no other medications.*

Oral Medication

If oral medication is desired:

1. chloral hydrate 50 mg/kg (maximum 2 g) with diphenhydramine 1.25 mg/kg (maximum 50 mg); *or*
2. for older children, diazepam, 5 to 10 mg.

Intramuscular Medication

If *intramuscular medication* is desired, the following combination works well for small bowel biopsy: meperidine 1 mg/kg (maximum 50 mg) and pentobarbital (Nembutal) 5 mg/kg (maximum 100 mg).

For Upper and Lower Gastrointestinal Endoscopy

Children

Intravenous diazepam and meperidine may be administered in a manner similar to the use in adults. Midazolam is a new benzodiazepine that is likely to replace diazepam as premedication for endoscopy in children; however, at the time of publication, the safety and effectiveness of this drug in children had not been established. Drugs are given slowly while observing the patient's cardiorespiratory status and level of sedation. Some children seem to become agitated with diazepam. In addition, the effects of meperidine are more easily reversed (with naloxone). Therefore, we tend to use relatively more meperidine. Meperidine is usually given in a dose from 1 to 2 mg/kg. Depending on the length of the procedure, the respiratory status, and the level of consciousness, as much as 3 to 4 mg/kg total dose of meperidine is given occasionally in smaller increments. As in adults, the diazepam dose should be carefully titrated. Children often require proportionately larger doses than adults; however, even in older children, one should probably not use more than 10 mg diazepam. If a child continues to be combative despite heavy sedation, it is safer to do the procedure under general anesthesia with the airway protected. This step is rarely necessary.

Infants

Infants almost never require general anesthesia when upper endoscopy is performed by an individual experienced in examining infants with the newer pediatric endoscopes. Infants under 6 months of age often tolerate upper endoscopy extremely well with no sedation. They object to swallowing the endoscope, but once passed, will often suck on the tube and fall asleep. Light sedation may be administered in this age group as necessary. Up to 2 to 3 years of age, it is usually simplest to administer sedation by mouth or intramuscularly. Beyond this age, intravenous administration allows one to titrate the quantity of drug against the requirements of the child.

Procedures in Infants and Children
Upper GI Endoscopy

Endoscopy may be performed with nearly any child from full-term newborn upward, using a pediatric endoscope. Only rarely will the instrument fail to pass through the pylorus in a young infant. Swabbing or spraying the posterior pharynx with local anesthetic can be helpful, but is not absolutely necessary. Biopsies are performed as in adults. Biopsies are especially helpful in evaluating esophagitis because gross appearance of the esophagus may be misleading, and symptoms are often vague in children. Foreign bodies can be removed from the upper GI tract with the use of grasping forceps or snare. This can be done under general anesthesia or with sedation and the use of an overtube.

Esophageal Dilatation

The indications and contraindications are similar to those in adults. The main limitation is the lack of cooperation that can occur when multiple dilatations are necessary. Ideally, if this is a problem, these dilatations can be done in an ambulatory surgery setting with brief anesthesia. Hurst and Maloney dilators are probably used most often in children; however, Gruentzig balloon dilatation can be performed in the same manner as in adults. With the use of the Gruentzig balloon, Puestow dilatations will probably be done much less frequently in children. The latter procedure requires the greatest amount of cooperation of all of these methods of dilatation.

Sclerotherapy for Esophageal Varices

Sclerotherapy can be performed in the same manner as in adults. Often this procedure can be done in children with intravenous sedation. If the child cannot remain quiet during the procedure, brief anesthesia may be necessary. Sclerotherapy can be performed in infants, although the volume of each injection probably should be reduced to about one-quarter of the adult dose. Early experience suggests that sclerotherapy may be especially beneficial for varices secondary to extrahepatic portal hypertension.

Percutaneous Liver Biopsy

The indications for liver biopsy in infants are somewhat different from those used in adults. The most common reason for liver biopsy in an infant is the evaluation of neonatal cholestasis. The differential diagnosis differs from that of cholestasis in adults. Therefore, the evaluation of these infants should only be done by a physician familiar with this differential and knowledgeable about the studies necessary. In older children, the most common indication for liver biopsy is chronic hepatitis. Although one cannot expect an infant or child to be cooperative for percutaneous liver biopsy, this procedure can be done safely if adequate sedation is given. As for adults, coagulation studies (including a bleeding time) should be checked before a biopsy is performed. After biopsy, the patient's vital signs should be monitored frequently. Having a patient lie on the right side for 2 hr after the biopsy and remain at bedrest until the next morning is standard procedure; however, it is often easiest to keep an infant or young child quiet and calm in his or her mother's arms.

An 18-gauge pediatric Menghini needle is available; however, many physicians who perform liver biopsies in infants and children prefer a No. 16 Menghini or Klatskin needle, since the No. 18 needle provides a specimen of less adequate width. The liver biopsy needle is longer than necessary for a child but may be used safely if it is held firmly between the thumb and forefinger 1.5 to 3 cm from the skin when the needle tip is at the liver surface. This provides a guard against excess penetration. The biopsy is performed at the midpoint of upper and lower dullness to percussion or may be performed subcostally if the liver is enlarged at least several centimeters below the costal margin. The procedure is similar to the method in adults, except that it is unrealistic to expect the patient to exhale on command. The biopsy can be timed with the respiratory cycle of the patient while the child is breathing quietly.

Rigid and Flexible Sigmoidoscopy

Specially designed rigid sigmoidoscopes of 11 mm diameter and 10 cm length are available for use in young infants; however, these instruments are rarely needed since the introduction of flexible sigmoidoscopy. This technique can be used in any age child except for very small neonates (under 1,500–

2,000 g), using the proper size instrument. In infants, it is possible to obtain an excellent view of the rectum and, at times, the sigmoid and descending colon as well, with the use of a pediatric upper endoscope inserted as a colonoscope. In children beyond 2 years of age, we tend to use an adult colonoscope for flexible sigmoidoscopy.

For infants, preparation of the colon is usually unnecessary. For older children, one can prepare with medicines from above or below. If the evaluation is for mucosal details (e.g., colitis), we prefer to prepare from above with magnesium citrate or milk of magnesia plus a laxative to stimulate emptying of the rectum both given the night before the procedure. Alternatively, a balanced electrolyte solution, as described below, can be used; however, it is usually unnecessary to put the child through the unpleasantness of this preparation for an examination limited to the rectosigmoid. The child has a clear liquid meal the night before and again for breakfast. A tap-water or saline solution enema may be adequate alone if the child has loose stools. A Fleet phosphate enema immediately before the procedure works well if the evaluation is for polyps and mucosal detail is not a concern.

Sedation is unnecessary in infants and older children if the examination is limited to the rectum alone; however, preschoolers often will not allow any procedure without sedation. For more extensive examination, sedation as described above for minor procedures is appropriate.

Colonoscopy and Polypectomy

Pediatric colonoscopes are available for use in young children, although an adult colonoscope can be used beyond the first year or two of age. Preparation of the colon is probably best done the night before the procedure with a balanced electrolyte solution given by mouth or nasogastric tube. Younger children will not voluntarily drink an adequate quantity of this solution, and the latter method is usually necessary. Nausea often accompanies the administration of this solution in children, and it is advisable to give metoclopramide (0.1 mg/kg) before the start. The proper volumes of these solutions for size have not been established. As a starting point, we use 1,000 ml/1.73 m^2/hr given over 3 to 4 hr; however, the solution should be continued until the stools are clear. Only clear liquids are allowed for supper and breakfast. Sedation is identical to that used for upper endoscopy, although intravenous sedation is often given at a younger age, since this procedure is associated with greater discomfort.

Most colonic polyps in children are juvenile polyps. These polyps tend to autoamputate and do not require routine removal. The indications for polypectomy include significant blood loss, abdominal pain, recurrent intussusception, prolapse, persistent rectal bleeding beyond 6 to 12 months, or removal for diagnostic purposes. However, colonoscopy is used frequently as a primary mode of evaluation of rectal bleeding, and polyps are often identified during this procedure. At that point it seems appropriate to perform a polypectomy even when the above criteria have not been met rather than have the possibility of doing a colonoscopy later for removal. In addition, parents are often relieved to have the polyp removed despite previous reassurance that it is benign. The method of polypectomy is identical to that used for adult patients.

Colonic Biopsy

Endoscopic biopsy of the colonic mucosa is performed in the same manner as in adults. Coagulation studies should be evaluated prior to biopsy. If a larger or deeper biopsy is required, e.g., for Hirschsprung's disease, suction biopsy can be done safely in any age infant or child, using a Rubin-Quinton tube (4,5). An adequate specimen to diagnose Hirschsprung's disease requires that the depth of submucosa be at least equal to the depth of the mucosa. Therefore, it has been recommended that 15 to 20 mm Hg pressure be applied when doing a suction biopsy for this diagnosis. The biopsy should be done above the distal 1 to 2 cm of rectum but below the peritoneal reflection. Ganglion cells are morphologically immature in infants in the first months of life and can best be identified by an experienced individual.

REFERENCES

1. Ament ME, Christie DL (1977): Upper gastrointestinal fiberoptic endoscopy in pediatric patients. *Gastroenterology* 72:1244–1248.
2. Andrassy RJ, Issacs H, Weitzman JJ (1981): Rectal suction biopsy for the diagnosis of Hirschsprung's disease. *Ann Surg* 193:419–424.
3. Cadranel S, Rodesch P, Peeters JP, Cremer M (1977): Fiberendoscopy of the gastrointestinal tract in children. *Am J Dis Child* 131:41–45.
4. Hargrove CB, Ulshen MH, Shub MD (1984): Upper gastrointestinal endoscopy in infants: diagnostic usefulness and safety. *Pediatrics* 74:828–831.
5. Howard ER, Stamatakis JD, Mowat AP (1984): Management of varices in children by injection sclerotherapy. *J Pediatr Surg* 19:2–5.
6. Shub MD, Ulshen MH, Hargrove CB, Siegal GP, Groben PA, Askin FA (1985): Esophagitis: a frequent consequence of gastroesophageal reflux in infancy. *J Pediatr* 107:881–884.
7. Vanderhoff JA, Ament ME (1976): Proctosigmoidoscopy and rectal biopsy in infants and children. *J Pediatr* 89:911–915.
8. Yunis EJ, Dibbins AW, Sherman FE (1976): Rectal suction biopsy in the diagnosis of Hirschsprung disease in infants. *Arch Pathol Lab Med* 100:329–333.

37 / Small Bowel Biopsy in Pediatric Patients

Martin H. Ulshen

In general, small bowel biopsy in a child is similar to biopsy in an adult. Usually, the Carey capsule or pediatric Crosby-Kugler capsule is quicker and easier to use in a child than the Rubin-Quinton tube. The Carey capsule is simplest, but the pediatric Crosby-Kugler capsule, which is shortest, occasionally passes through the pylorus in a young infant (less than 1 month of age) when the Carey capsule will not.

Indications

1. Diagnosis of any of the diffuse mucosal diseases of small intestine (e.g., gluten sensitive enteropathy, eosinophilic gastroenteritis, abeta-lipoproteinemia).
2. Confirmation of disaccharidase deficiency (e.g., congenital sucrase-isomaltase deficiency).
3. Diagnosis of Giardia when stool specimens are negative.

Contraindications

1. Bleeding disorder (see Chapter 23, Contraindications, item 2).
2. Severe malnutrition with hypoproteinemia and/or hypokalemia.

Preparation

1. Older children should be given nothing by mouth overnight; in young infants, give nothing by mouth for 4 hr only.

2. Sedation may be required in patients up to 6 to 8 years of age and may be given as needed in older children. Pre-medications may be given p.o. or i.m. (see Chapter 36).
3. Topical anesthesia may be used in patients who are not sedated.
4. Check hematocrit, platelet count, PT, PTT.
5. Explain procedure to family and to child as well, if old enough to understand.

Equipment

1. Carey capsule with cardiac catheter tubing and cardiac catheter straight guide wire (or Crosby-Kugler capsule with similar tubing).
2. Outer bite protection tubing. This is a 10- to 15-cm length of No. 14 French nasogastric tubing that has a longitudinal slit (cut with scissors). This tubing can be placed over the more delicate cardiac catheter tubing for protection during swallowing and can be subsequently removed without disassembly of the capsule and cardiac catheter tubing.
3. Fluoroscope.
4. Suction.
5. Plastic mesh.
6. Forceps.
7. Fine scissors.
8. Aluminum foil.
9. Glass slides.

Procedure

1. Assemble the capsule.
2. Test the capsule.

   a. Carey—be sure the spring is in place and that the capsule moves freely.
   b. Crosby—place rubber glove against ports and trigger with syringe.

3. It is best to swaddle a child who may be uncooperative in addition to providing sedation. Children over 5 to 8 years of age frequently will not require these measures.

4. With the guide wire and outer plastic bite tubing in place, pass the capsule to the posterior pharynx. It is easiest with an uncooperative child to start with the child or infant lying supine. Maintain steady, light pressure on the outer tube and pass this as the child swallows.

5. Once the capsule is in the esophagus, withdraw the outer bite tube and keep the cardiac catheter tubing against the buccal mucosa with an index finger. Be sure your finger is far enough into the mouth to keep the tube away from the molars. If this is done correctly (and an assistant holds the child's head still), the child cannot bite you or the tubing. Older children may prefer to hold the tubing themselves.

6. Rotate the child to lie on the right side and advance the tubing. Fluoroscope in 1-sec bursts to observe the position of the capsule. It may be necessary to shake an infant up and down gently to have the capsule fall toward the pylorus.

7. Adjust the tubing to position the capsule in the region of the pylorus and apply steady, moderate pressure to the tubing. If the capsule does not pass through the pylorus easily, manipulate the abdomen with a gloved hand to help move the capsule through. A thumb under the capsule pushing cephalad or under the loop of the tubing along the greater curvature may change the relationship of the capsule with the pylorus and allow it to pass through. If there is difficulty, several cubic centimeters of ice water may be passed through to stimulate the antrum to contract and pop the capsule through the pylorus. Metoclopramide premedication is not absolutely necessary but can speed up the positioning of the capsule. The dose of metoclopramide is 0.1 mg/kg and can be given orally.

8. Once the capsule has entered the second portion of the duodenum, it may move more quickly if the guide wire is pulled back several centimeters or removed completely.

9. For the Carey capsule: After removal of the guide wire, duodenal contents may be aspirated with light, steady pressure. When this is complete, wash capsule through with about 3 to 5 cc water followed by a similar amount

of air. Move the capsule slightly so that mucosa traumatized during aspiration is not at the port. The biopsy is usually taken at the ligament of Treitz. If the Crosby-Kugler capsule is used, a second tubing may be placed over or alongside the cardiac catheter tubing to allow aspiration of fluid. However, fluid cannot be aspirated through the biopsy capsule.

10. To close the Carey capsule, use a 50-ml syringe and apply steady, firm pressure. You can see the capsule close with fluoroscopy. Syringe pressure must be maintained to keep it closed. To close the Crosby-Kugler capsule, pull on the syringe plunger sharply several times.

11. An assistant can remove the tubing and capsule with steady pressure, always being sure the child cannot bite the tubing.

12. When pressure is released, the Carey capsule will pop open, and the biopsy will be on the spring with mucosal side down. The Crosby-Kugler capsule must be opened to retrieve the two biopsy specimens obtained. You can spread the biopsy by gently teasing with the side of a needle. The specimen will tend to curl up with mucosal side out. Mount mucosa side up on plastic mesh and, if necessary, spread biopsy again. (This is easiest to do if mesh is lying on a glass slide.) With fine scissors, cut off specimen(s) if needed for enzyme assay. Specimens for disaccharidase assay may be frozen for later analysis. A mucus touch prep for Giardia can be obtained by gently touching the biopsy specimen or the Carey capsule spring to a glass slide and immediately placing this slide into fixative for cytologic processing.

Postprocedure

1. Place a brief note in the patient's record that includes the type of procedure, studies for which specimen saved, and amount of fluoroscopy time.

2. When the child is alert, he or she may drink clear liquids and may eat or drink $\frac{1}{2}$ hr later if topical anesthesia has worn off.

3. The patient may leave the hospital 2 to 3 hr after biopsy if he or she lives within 1- to 2-hr drive.

REFERENCES

1. Carey JB (1964): A simplified gastrointestinal biopsy capsule. *Gastroenterology* 46:550–557.
2. Kilby A (1976): Paediatric small intestinal biopsy capsule with two ports. *Gut* 17:158–159.

38 / Breath Hydrogen Test

Martin H. Ulshen

The breath hydrogen (H_2) test is a simple, noninvasive study for carbohydrate intolerance that is easily performed. It can be used for infants and children as well as adults. The test is extremely sensitive and, in fact, identifies individuals with asymptomatic carbohydrate malabsorption. For this reason, the results must be interpreted in the context of the clinical setting.

Indications

1. Detection of carbohydrate intolerance, most commonly a disaccharidase deficiency.
2. Diagnosis of bacterial overgrowth.

Contraindications

None.

Preparation

1. Test for carbohydrate intolerance. Patient should be given nothing by mouth overnight (a minimum of 4–6 hr in infants).
2. Test for bacterial overgrowth. Measure breath H_2 after an overnight fast; the previous night's dinner should be meat and rice bread (avoid other starches).
3. Patient should not be on antibiotics at the time of study.

Equipment

1. Breath H_2 analyzer.
2. Breath-sampling device and collection bags.

Procedure

Collection of Breath Samples

Breath samples can be collected with a nasal cannula in an infant or with a mouthpiece and a one-way valve in a child or adult. Collection in infants is timed to manually sample several expirations with the use of a syringe.

Test for Carbohydrate Intolerance

1. A baseline breath sample is collected before administering the carbohydrate.
2. The patient then drinks a 10% to 20% aqueous solution of the carbohydrate under study (1–2 g/kg; maximum of 50 g).
3. Breath samples are collected at intervals of at least 30 min for $1\frac{1}{2}$ to 2 hr; these samples can be analyzed at the time of collection or saved and analyzed simultaneously.

Test for Bacterial Overgrowth

A single fasting sample is collected.

Postprocedure

Return to previous activities.

Complications

Diarrhea secondary to carbohydrate intolerance.

Interpretation

Carbohydrate Intolerance

Although interpretation of this test is not standardized, most often a rise in H_2 above baseline of greater than 10 to 20 ppm is considered abnormal.

Bacterial Overgrowth

A fasting breath H_2 of greater than 11 ppm is considered abnormal.

REFERENCES

1. Ostrander CR, Cohen RS, Hopper AO, et al (1983): Breath hydrogen analysis: a review of the methodologies and clinical applications. *J Pediatr Gastroenterol Nutr* 2:525–533.
2. Perman JA, Barr RG, Watkins JB (1978): Sucrose malabsorption in children: noninvasive diagnosis by interval breath hydrogen determination. *J Pediatr* 93:17–22.
3. Perman JA, Modler S, Barr RG (1984): Fasting breath hydrogen concentration: normal values and clinical application. *Gastroenterology* 87:1358–1363.
4. Levitt MD, Bond JH (1981): Quantitative measurement of lactose absorption and colonic salvage of nonabsorbed lactose: direct and indirect methods. In: *Lactose Digestion: Clinical and Nutritional Implications*, edited by DM Paige and TM Bayless, pp 80–87. The Johns Hopkins University Press, Baltimore.
5. Solomons NW (1981): Diagnosis and screening techniques for lactose maldigestion: advantages of the hydrogen breath test. In: *Lactose Digestion: Clinical and Nutritional Implications*, edited by DM Paige and TM Bayless, pp 91–109. The Johns Hopkins University Press, Baltimore.
6. Barr RG (1981): Limitations of the hydrogen breath test and other techniques for predicting incomplete lactose absorption. In: *Lactose Digestion: Clinical and Nutritional Implications*, edited by DM Paige and TM Bayless, pp 110–114. The Johns Hopkins University Press, Baltimore.

39 / Esophageal pH Monitoring for Gastroesophageal Reflux

Martin H. Ulshen

Esophageal pH can be monitored to evaluate the presence of gastroesophageal reflux (GER). There are two major methods of monitoring: a continuous, extended study or a brief study (Tuttle test; see also Chapter 6). The former method appears to be more reliable. Monitoring requires adequate cooperation to maintain a pH probe in the esophagus for the duration of the study; however, the newer ambulatory monitoring systems allow the patient to continue normal activities during study. Perhaps the greatest weakness in this test is the wide variability in the methods of analyzing the results.

Indications

1. Confirmation of questionable esophageal symptoms or sequelae of GER.
2. Evaluation for the presence of GER in patients with chronic lung disease or recurrent apnea.

Contraindications

None.

Preparation

Patient should be given nothing by mouth for at least 4 hr prior to passing the pH probe.

Equipment

1. Flexible pH microelectrode.
2. Device for measuring and recording pH:
   a. pH meter with recording terminals, patient isolator, strip chart recorder; or
   b. ambulatory pH meter with microprocessor recording device, microcomputer (or dedicated microprocessor), and printer.

Procedure

1. If necessary, the pH meter is calibrated against buffer (pH 4.0 and 7.0) before inserting the probe.
2. Following application of a local anesthetic solution to the nasal mucosa (4% cocaine works well), the pH probe is passed nasally under fluoroscopic control. The probe is passed into the stomach to document an acid pH and then pulled back to the distal esophagus in the region of the mid-left atrium. The probe should always be at least 2.5 cm above the gastroesophageal junction. The probe lead is immobilized by taping it to the nose at the external naris.
3. *Tuttle test.* A volume of 0.1 N HCl adjusted for size (300 ml/1.73 m^2) is given to the patient through a nasogastric tube. Alternatively, apple juice can be given orally in a volume appropriate for size. Esophageal pH is monitored for 10 min with the patient prone or lying on a side. If no GER is seen, abdominal pressure is increased by manual compression, valsalva, crying, and straight-leg raising for 5 to 10 min.
4. *Extended study.* Recording is done over a period of 12 to 24 hr. The patient maintains a chronologic log of activities, including position (upright, supine, prone); sleep times; mealtimes; and other events (regurgitation, coughing, heartburn, etc.).
5. If a pH meter is used, the meter reading should be re-checked against pH 4.0 buffer at the end of the study.
6. If an ambulatory system is used, the data is fed from the ambulatory microprocessor unit into the computer or dedicated microprocessor.

Postprocedure

Normal diet and activities.

Complications

Virtually none; very low risk of aspiration, as with a small-caliber feeding tube.

Interpretation

Has not been well standardized.

Tuttle Test

Two or more episodes of pH <4.0 for >15 sec apiece is a positive result.

Evaluation of Extended pH Study

There are at least three methods for evaluating the extended pH study.

1. Reflux is defined as an episode with pH <4.0 that lasts at least 15 sec. A weighted score is given for the number of episodes per 12 hr; number of episodes greater than 5 min in duration per 12 hr; longest episode, and total percent of time with esophageal pH <4.0 during periods awake, asleep, upright, and supine. A final score is derived and compared to an upper limit of normal.
2. Pathologic GER is defined as pH <4.0 for greater than 10% of the postprandial period.
3. Pathologic GER is defined as pH <4.0 for greater than 4 min, or a mean of more than 1.5 episodes with pH <4.0, per hour.

REFERENCES

1. Euler AR, Ament ME (1977): Detection of gastroesophageal reflux in the pediatric-age patient by esophageal intraluminal pH probe measurement (Tuttle test). *Pediatrics* 60:65–68.
2. Jolley SG, Johnson DG, Herbst JJ, et al (1978): An assessment of

gastroesophageal reflux in children by extended pH monitoring of the distal esophagus. *Surgery* 84:16–24.

3. Sondheimer JM (1980): Continuous monitoring of distal esophageal pH: a diagnostic test for gastroesophageal reflux in infants. *J Pediatr* 96:804–807.

4. Winter HS, Madara JL, Stafford RJ, et al (1982): Intraepithelial eosinophils: a new diagnostic criterion for reflux esophagitis. *J Pediatr* 83:818–823.

Subject Index

Colitis, pseudomembranous,
120
Collagen disease, 86
"Colon coagulation
syndrome," 228
Colonic biopsy, in pediatric
patients, 241
Colonoscopic polypectomy,
223–229
complications of, 228–229
contraindications for, 223
equipment for, 223
indication for, 223
in pediatric patients, 240–
241
postprocedure for, 228
preparation for, 223–224
procedure for, 224–228
Colonoscopy, 110–118
contraindications for, 111
equipment for, 113
indications for, 110–111
in pediatric patients, 240–
241
postprocedure for, 117–118
preparation for, 111–113
procedure for, 113–117
Contraction(s)
external sphincter, 83
tertiary, in esophageal body,
39,43
Culture, in percutaneous liver
biopsy, 153
Cytology
pancreatic, 107–108
in percutaneous liver
biopsy, 153
in upper GI endoscopy, 95

D

Decompression, endoscopic
biliary, *see* Endoscopic
biliary decompression

Descending colon, 116
Diagnosis
of exocrine pancreatic
insufficiency, 136–139
of gastrinoma, 133–135
of pernicious anemia, 60
of Zollinger-Ellison
syndrome, 59–60
Diagnostic indications, for
upper GI endoscopy, 90
Diagnostic paracentesis, 142–
144
Diffuse esophageal spasm, 41
Digital examination, 128–129
Dilatation
balloon, *see* Balloon
dilatation
esophageal, *see* Esophageal
dilatation
Direct gastric placement, of
feeding tubes, 12–13
Direct heat thermal cautery,
231
Disease
collagen, 86
inflammatory bowel, 120
Disorder(s)
of external sphincter
dysfunction, 86–87
muscle versus nervous, 87
Duodenal aspiration, 77–79
complications of, 78
indications for, 72
endoscopically assisted,
78–79
Duodenum
placement of feeding tubes
into
endoscopically guided,
13–14
by gravity, 13
visualization of, in upper GI
endoscopy, 93